MW01171619

Health, Humor, and a Hole in the Wall

*Dealing with Health Challenges and
Aging from a Humorous Perspective*

By Jim LeDuc

"LeDuc's book, "Health, Humor, and a Hole in the Wall" is a must read for any man, and for the women that love them. It chronicles the Murphy's Law of what can go wrong with a man's health after 40. A hilariously good read! Laugh out-loud funny (Do not attempt to read this in a quiet place!). This is the only book I've ever finished
"cover to cover" in one sitting!"

Julie Cooley

"Once in a while, you run across a book that you can't put down. Belly laughter is a friend of mine who I don't hear from all that often anymore. People from southern California that have had as many surgeries as Jim usually don't look the same as when they began exchanging skin for plastic. I found myself unable to put this book down until its end, enjoyed the company of my long-lost friend, belly laughter, and believe that after splitting my side from reading Jim's book, that I may be in need some surgical procedure myself! Not sure how a guy who has a body that hurts so much, for so long, has been able to stay sane enough, and keep his sense of humor intact and be able to relay such a refreshing story. Glad he was able, and
I think you will be, too."

John Lane, Santiago High School

"Jim LeDuc's book, *Health, Humor, and a Hole in the Wall* is a must read for the old and young alike. Through his own personal journey of aging and the medical mishaps he encounters along the way, the reader is taken on a humorous adventure that will leave them laughing out loud and wanting more. Through his down-to-earth, speak from the heart style, the reader is able to grasp his message of overcoming obstacles and living each day to the fullest without feeling preached to. Jim's ability to turn lemons into lemonade at every turn of his own life inspires readers to reevaluate their own life struggles and see them from a new, positive perspective."

Stephanie Ransom

"Jim LeDuc's humor is as quick and abrupt as his reactions to the wide variety of medical procedures and after effects that his body has sustained. The narrative that takes us through every conceivable part of Jim's anatomy is not for the squeamish but is for the majority of us who have been subjected to the humiliation of a medical exam or procedure. His descriptions cut into your funny bone like a scalpel, making it impossible not to laugh and to be thankful that it is Jim going through the insanity, not the reader. One walks away from the book surprised the Jim is still upright, but happy that he has written his thoughts down."

Nathan Theune

"It would be impossible to avoid aging. Health, Humor and a Hole makes laughing possible while getting old."

Lupe Aguirre

"Jim (LeDuc) paints quite an amusing picture of what we may all go through as we gracefully age! If laughter is indeed a healing quality, then the reader has a head start in staying healthy. If he/she isn't fortunate enough to avoid some of the aging pitfalls, then forewarned is forearmed. Behind the humor of this book is a positive approach to life in general and health in specific that we all can benefi t from."

Pat Smith

"Jim LeDuc is the man. His book Health, Humor, and a Hole in the Wall is a hilarious look at aging and myriad of physiological failures that await us all. As a colleague of Jim's, I expected nothing less from the man who has always been genuine and open to all of us here on campus. However, his writing touches not only those of us who either are experiencing the same symptoms of aging, or are close, but is relevant to those that have also faced other health challenges in their lives as well. I purchased a copy for my son, Jimmy, who is now twenty-three and a former student of Jim's. As a young boy, Jimmy faced his own health issues. Our family found that humor and a positive outlook on the realities of illness were the only way to survive the otherwise mind-numbing reality of disease. After reading the book, Jimmy and I both feel we have a comrade in arms with Jim. If you feel that life is getting you down and the only luck that you seem to have is bad luck, then pick up a copy of Health, Humor and a Hole in the Wall for a comical look at reality. Sometimes insanity is a good thing!"

Tami Lincoln, Teacher, Santiago High School

Contents

Prologue 6

Chapter 1..8
The Symptoms of Aging or You Know That You Are Gtting Old When

Chapter 2 23
The Two "Cystas," Pilonidal and Blood

Chapter 3 28
The Knees: Snap, Crackle, Pop, or Klunk

Chapter 4 33
The Double Hernia, Balls in a Vice Grip, Bowel-Imprisoned Air Pockets, or The Great Migration

Chapter 5 46
IVs, Transfusions, Catheters, and Jumbo Wipes

Chapter 6 108
A Colonoscopy Is Kind of Like a NASA Apollo Moon Launch

Chapter 7..122
Lower Back Pain, Surgeries, and Pain Management or An Israelite's Perspective of Wandering in the Wilderness for Forty Years

Chapter 8 174
Aging and Urination. A Delicate Topic for Delicate Times

Chapter 9 195
So My Health Is Shot. What Do I Do Now?

Chapter 10...214
As a Dog Returns to Its Vomit…

.

Prologue

I think that I have a right and an obligation to write my story—or at least my story up until now. The end of my story is still yet to happen, although I have a pretty good picture of how it is going to end up. That is, if my medical history since I turned 40 is any indication of how my next 25 years will go, then I have yet to experience 32 surgical procedures. That means that if I do survive the next 25 years, which is entirely possible as advanced medicine has prolonged human life considerably over the past 50 years, then I will still only be 77 years of age which is not really that old by today's standards. Yet if I do make it 25 more years and 33 more surgeries, then I will have had 50 surgical procedures since the age of 40! Certainly, if that does indeed happen, then I will have to be considered for at least an honorable mention in the Guinness Book of World Records for most surgical procedures due to aging and not a severe accident of some kind!

Don't get me wrong. I do want to be around to see my children all marry and to bounce my grandchildren on my knee—even if there is no cartilage—but I want to enjoy the ride. Heck, I even want to be around to see my grandkids grow up and I want to take them fishing and on cruises and all the other grandpa-grandkid stuff. But, I have no desire to have them push me around in a wheelchair while I wonder who these nice people are and when my next bowl of oatmeal will be served as long as it is no later than 4:30 in the afternoon which will be my bedtime!

Maybe I am getting ahead of myself. Permit me to back up and explain what I mean. My age as of this writing is 52 years.

Since I turned 40, I have had 17 surgical procedures besides all of the standard probes and pricks (no reference to any of my doctors who may be reading this) including the main list of procedures as follows: 1 thumb, 1 Lasik procedure (on both eyes), 2 cysts surgically removed, 3 knee surgeries, 2 hernias including one side and then a repeat along with the other side, 4 back, 1 gall bladder, and 1 colonoscopy (saving the best for last!).

Now there might be someone out there that has had way more surgical procedures than I have, but the stories behind some of these surgical procedures are the inspiration for writing this personal history.

Before I get started, I would like to establish a few key points. First, I have good insurance. If you were to add up the cost of all of these procedures, they would add up to about a million dollars—and that is certainly no joke! Next, these stories are all true. I may take just a little bit of literary license, but the events contained herein are all factual. Finally, I would like to express my gratitude to all the medical staff that have taken part in my experiences and I would like to express my love for my dear wife who has stood by my side—and my bedside—with undeviating love and support. To her, I dedicate this book.

Chapter 1

The Symptoms of Aging or You Know That You Are Getting Old When…

Once I hit that magical age of 40 and even a bit before that, I began to experience some symptoms of aging. For those of you younger guys out there, let this be a voice of warning. And for all you ladies who dare to read this, you need to understand that when your man begins to experience some of these symptoms, then he is getting old and you need to start facing the reality of that fact. Remember that ignoring these symptoms does not cause them to disappear and even though there are medical breakthroughs that can disguise or even temporarily take these symptoms away, once the aging process begins, there is no going back. No matter what you say, how you act, or what you drive, you are still aging.

To put this in better perspective, let me explain the process like this: I am a schoolteacher of psychology. I am not a biologist. My strength in psychology is in the field of behavior, not biology or neuroscience. In psychology, we do study some physiology. We even delve into the different developmental stages of life from infancy to old age. I have learned through my experience in teaching this field one simple fact: Throughout life, our cells are constantly regenerating themselves. But, as we get older, our cells no longer are able to replenish themselves and as they die off, new cells do not grow back. This means that quite literally, we begin to decompose right before our very own eyes and there isn't a damn thing we can do about it!

As I think of some of the symptoms that begin to show up to let us know that the old biological clock is ticking, I thought that perhaps I could present them much as David Letterman would do on his Late Show. And so, including a bit more detail than Dave would do, and in the form of self-reflective questions for personal or spousal evaluation, I give you my top ten signs of getting old—from a male perspective of course:

Sign Number 1:

Do big thick black hairs and even big thick albino and almost horse-like hairs grow out of your nose? And, when they do sprout up, and you do proceed to remove them with excruciating pain and eye-watering removal by a very primitive yanking out of the hair at the root—especially the hairs that grow on the very sensitive portion of the center of the nose—they amazingly are fully grown back the very next day?

I will say that there is some amazing but unfortunately temporary relief from the discomfort, breathe-blocking, and self-consciousness of nasal hair. My daughter is a cosmetologist. Her education was quite expensive and yet she decided to go back to school and get her Associate's Degree instead of working full time in her newly acquired vocation (by the way, I do believe in a college education as I have dual bachelor's degrees and a master's degree). However, through her cosmetology experience, she learned how to do facial waxing. Included in her waxing education is the knowledge of how to wax a man's nose! Now this is quite a process so let me explain it briefly—non-scientifically of course and without the use of all proper vocabulary words in the field of facial hair removal. First, you apply hot wax to the little stick. Next, you put the stick up the guy's nose. You must stick the stick up far enough to get to the top of the nasal cavity at about the end of the cartilage and the beginning of the nose bone. Then, you press the nose so that the opening of the nose closes around the stick. Next, you let dry for about two to three minutes. Finally, the person doing the hair removal places one open hand firmly against the forehead of the person receiving the waxing as she firmly grabs the stick with her other hand. And here is where the procedure gets a bit cloudy because I believe that there is a moment of temporary unconsciousness. She says, "On three," and begins counting, only instead of counting to three when you can fully brace yourself for the pain, she yanks the stick out on the count of two! And even though the pain is quite intense for a brief moment, the payoff is well worth the cost of the waxing, or in my case, the cost of the education. At that moment of euphoria, a guy is able to take a breath of fresh air by breathing out of his nose with the mouth entirely closed! And for a few brief number of days, this guy can breathe through his nose without any nasal cavity follicle interference and that...my friends is a truly liberating experience—especially when a guy has had to use mouth-assisted breathing for a number of years!

Sign Number 2:

Speaking of hair, do those same big, thick, black and coarse white hairs grow out of the inside of your ear or more embarrassingly, out of the middle of your ear lobe? Those hairs out the lobe sprout roots that are really tough to pull out. In fact, when you pull on these, your whole earlobe moves forward and it takes six to eight tries until you can dislodge the roots and pull the hair all of the way out! And if you're not careful, if you don't grab the hair at the skin line when you yank on it, you tear off the hair so that it protrudes out of the lobe just below the height needed to grab onto the hair to finish the deed so that the hair survives another day.

Sign Number 3:

This is the last thing that I will say about hair but I have to bring one more up since it is a sure sign of aging. Do your eyebrows continue to grow out regardless of the length, and once they reach a certain length, do they sort of frizz out and look like curly fries? And, does the rest of you body hair continue to grow longer and longer and longer like the hair on your chest, arms, legs, and genital area? If so, you are getting old!

I am amazed at all of the hair left in the sink when I trim my eyebrows! I used to use my facial razor and just shave up. But now that they have become curly fries, I have been forced to use a comb to stand them up and then trim them with some very sharp scissors. Otherwise, if the scissors are not very sharp, the eye brow hair just bends inside the blades instead of being cut off.

As far as the chest, arm and leg hair goes, I have seen some people that could actually braid the hair on their arms! Mine are not that bad—at least not yet anyway. For now, every once in a while, I will be sitting in my lounge chair watching television when the light of the TV reflects off of a hair that stands alone amongst the forest. This hair defies gravity and seems to go on forever. When I do come across one of these, I hate to pull it out. It is kind of like one of those trophies that you have had on the shelf for a long time that really aren't that important, but you still get some sort of satisfaction in looking at them and even taking them off the shelf and holding them every once in a while. So, I try not to pull it out even though the urge is quite strong. If I can withstand the temptation to pull it out, then when I get the opportunity, or when I remember that it is there, I can gently grab and extend it outward away from the skin and pet it. This can sort of be compared to a security blanket or your favorite slippers. There is just something soothing and comforting about having a very long, solitary hair around!

Getting back to Psychology and the aging process, we have also learned that sensory and nerve functioning begins to deteriorate as we get older. This is the source of the next several signs that let you know that you are getting old.

Sign Number 4:

This sign is quite frustrating and difficult to confess, yet it is most certainly a warning beacon to let you know that you are advancing in years. In my youth, I always tried to have good table manners. I always have a napkin in my hand or lap, and as I have aged, I usually have several extra ones within a hand's reach. And yet, even though I try to proceed with caution as I eat, inevitably I end up with someone pointing out that there is some food on my lips or somewhere in the vicinity of my mouth. The worst part is that I almost always have to change my shirt after I eat! I feel that I need to call out a CSI to determine the origin of the stains and how they got to some of the crazy locations where they end up. Frankly, I am getting tired of people—either politely by friends or acquaintances, or mockingly by immediate family members like my kids or wife or sister-in-law, pointing out the particles of food left on my face and staining my shirt! Now I realize that over the years my waist line has expanded and that more food will now end up on my shirt rather than pass through the ever-narrowing gap between my belly and the table, but that doesn't mean that the pill gets easier to swallow or the acceptance of the condition becomes easier to take. It just simply means that it does happen.

Sign Number 5:

Have you ever heard the one about the guy who while in the company of several friends brags that he just farted and yet no one heard it and it doesn't smell, and then his friends respond by telling him that he needs to go and see the ear and nose specialist? Well, that is aging my friends. Passing gas is just a part of life. Kids laugh at it, younger men brag about it, women try to ignore the subject altogether, and old people just really just don't care anymore! This then, is the point at which you know you are getting old—when you push it out, you think that since you didn't hear it, then no one else can even though it sounded something like starting up a chainsaw that just can't quite sustain the power because it is running on gas fumes. Furthermore, you can't smell it and so you think that no one else can either even though it mushrooms out quite similarly to an atomic blast, leaving a path of destruction that calls for immediate action of containment by the Hazmat team! And so after the act, you continue on your merry way feeling quite satisfied and accomplished, while oblivious to the swath of destruction that you have just laid out! At that point, you're literally an old fart! Enough said.

Sign Number 6:

When you are shaving or you perform that rare body examination which takes place spontaneously before you have a chance to catch yourself—even though you avoid looking at all mirrors and any reminders that gravity is taking effect and that you are drooping, sagging, swaying, and/or giggling, do you find three dimensional, misshapen, often discolored growths that seem to grow out of nowhere into the Rock of Gibraltar? Then you, my friend, are getting old!

When I was younger, I never had moles or weird looking growths of any kind. I just had zits like most puberty-passing teenagers. Now, I am completely caught off guard by the sheer numbers and the scary features of all these Wicked Witch of Any Compass Direction moles that crop up out of nowhere and in Olympic-magnitude record times! Without any warning much like the plagues of the Dark Ages, these things appear in all of their asymmetrical majesty in not only the most exposed parts of your face and upper body, but they also blossom out in the most obscure and isolated outposts in the human geographic anatomical atlas.

Of course, you can go to the doctor and get them burned off as I have done on several different occasions, but the problem is that once you begin the process of removal and much like an infestation of sewer rats, you can never keep up with the repopulation of the species. Further, it appears as if these apparitions grow stronger and even build up a sort of biological resistance against any and all treatments! All you can do is remove the gross ones, make sure that you never have a visible one that has hairs growing out of it, and make sure that you get them checked out often to ensure that none of them gains too much momentum! Remember this: don't get all excited about the suspicious ones before going to the doctor—relax! 99% of the time, the ones that look like Quasimodo end up being the most harmless!

Sign Number 7:

Scientific research has shown that human tissue continues to grow after death. However, have you noticed as you get older that you nose and ears start to grow again, only this time, unlike infancy and childhood development, your body growth has completely stopped so that these features will be forever enlarged and ultimately grotesquely disfigured? I shudder to reflect upon this very disturbing subject any longer, and so I will move on. Just accept one simple truth regarding this topic. As you age, your ears and nose just keep on growing and there is nothing you can do about it!

Sign Number 8:

Throughout adolescence and early adulthood, our physiques look pretty good. We are more muscular and fi rm. And, our skin fi ts our frame quite snugly. So with that being said as an intro, you know what is coming next. Now I am not going to ask if you have wrinkles because that would be too easy. We all have wrinkles. The question guys, is this: No matter how much you work out and take care of your body, when you move your head from side to side, does your neck trail behind? And when it does catch up with your face, does it wiggle like a bowl of Jell-O? Then you my friend (I keep calling you that—maybe because by now we have so much in common!) have JNS (Jiggle-Neck Syndrome), and unfortunately, there is no cure. Yes, you can temporarily halt the spreading of this progressive condition through face lifts or neck lifts, but you simply can't continue to stretch your face like that. How do you know when to quit you may ask? Well, when your eyes are looking directly ahead at the noon day sun and your ears touch at the back of your head, then it's time to give in.

The sad part about Jiggle-Neck Syndrome is that ultimately, your neck begins to show signs that Darwin really did know what he was talking about as we begin to look more and more like our ornithological ancestors, the turkey and the buzzard!

Sign Number 9:

This sign took me totally off-guard as I ignorantly ASS-umed that it only occurred with my friend who is ten years older than me—so prepare yourself! No matter how many times you wash your hair in a day, do you wake up in the morning with the top of your head smelling like the exhale of a decomposing corpse who has just been dredged up out of the depths of a stagnate lake? Does your pillow stink like grandpa's underwear and you know for a fact that he only sports one pair? Does the headrest of your favorite lounge chair smell like the remains left behind in your backyard pooper-scooper? Then you my friend are now cursed for the rest of your mortal existence with the notorious Morning Stink-Head! This may be the most traumatic of all of the symptoms because when you suddenly and without any warning whatsoever find yourself with it, you have a strong urge to go find a self-help book on taking scalps, get a very sharp Ginsu knife, and try to cut it out like you would a very aggressive, non-curable cancer. But don't try this as unfortunately science has proven that stink-head originates much, much further than skin deep.

Sign Number 10:

I would say that perhaps I have saved the best for last but that would be like saying that I saved you the best piece of chicken— the gizzard. Or, it may even be like telling you that I have just set you up on a real hot blind date only to find out that you are stuck with the very nicest, most kind and caring gall in the movie Shallow Hal. Anyway you slice it, brace yourself 'cause here it comes and I really do not have any delicate way of presenting this question. It could be compared to, "Did you know that you really are the bastard son of a serial killer on death row?" Or, "Did I happen to mention to you that I saw your wife's name, photograph and e-mail address on a web site entitled America's Most Promiscuous?"

Well, I have delayed it long enough. I cannot put it delicately or sugarcoat it so without further ado, here is the question regarding the 10th sign of getting old: Have your testicles dropped? Do they do nothing more than bump and bounce together as you walk along in your leisure wear? Then you are suffering from what I call Clackeritis. Put simply, your little buddies are like Clackers on a string that clack back and forth like that cheap old toy that we got in the 60's with the two glassy balls on a string.

Now if you are still in denial about this, ask yourself these two questions: Can you compare the space that your little guys have in their quaint little studio apartment like trying to sleep in a mummy bag inside a one-man pup tent? Or, is it more like they're snoozing on a hammock on a lazy afternoon? Do your old friends get wet when you sit down on the toilet? Then face the facts. You my friend are old!

Alternate Sign (in case you have a rare sort of immunity to one of the above which is actually called denial and you better accept it and deal with it!):

The male gender has been provided with different plumbing than the females of our species. As I have aged, my doctor refers to it as my pipe works. As part of this complex system of fluid flow, hydraulics, and propagation of the species multi-task functioning, there is a symbolic master valve or steam generator we call the prostate. I am not going to give you an anatomy lesson and certainly if you are male and over the age of 50, your prostate has been checked and rechecked as has mine. Although I have been shown its location on a doctor's office poster, I am still not exactly sure where this little gadget is located. However, I believe that it is located somewhere south of the border between Baja California and Mexico City. As far as the male aging process is concerned, I guess that what I am trying to say in a tactful way and in an attempt to defend my manliness and macho image is that somewhere down the road to duffer-hood, a man's hot rod or vehicle he just loves to drive and which brings him great pleasure and intense excitement, starts to have some mechanical problems and break down more and more frequently. In other words, as a man gets older, his mechanical operations start to get old and worn out and he sort of loses his killer instinct or "drive" for perpetuating mankind and is forced into retirement. No longer can he just jump in the car and go for a ride. Rather, he ends up parking the old companion in the garage and is forced to get around town by purchasing a city bus pass. Bottom line— his once voracious appetite for sensuality has now been replaced with the satisfaction of a good movie and a large bowl of ice cream.

Speaking of the good old water works, when I went to see my doctor for my 50-year-old checkup, I was given some homework and assigned tutoring. First, I had to get my cholesterol checked along with some other blood work. I'm no medical expert, but I have a theory that men started to die off prematurely from cholesterol, high blood pressure, plaque built up clogged arteries, and a myriad of other internal mal-functioning, only after we started to take all these tests. Before doctors ordered all these blood, urine, tissue, stools, and other bodily fluid tests, men were fi ne. Now that we have to donate part of our innermost being every time we go in for a check-up, or even just the fact that each time we are pricked or probed in a medical facility, part of our natural immunities is tainted somehow. Or every time we older guys go in for a checkup, we are given a plethora of symptoms, conditions, and health risks so extensive, they play on our brain and we are so caught up in the thought of all these problems, our bodies are faked into believing we are going to die and so we do! I think that we were just fi ne and that the average life span of a typical male would be at least ten years longer if the doctors would have just let us alone. Now days, once we turn 50, we are now predestined to be labeled with multiple conditions that are certain to bring about our early demise. (Just a thought I have)

Back to my check up, I also got a referral to go and have a colonoscopy done. Now I had heard a little about this, but little did I know—right? Anyway, this story is reserved as a chapter of it's own. In the results of my blood work, there was some evidence of an enlarged prostate (those little blood cell sellout bastards!) and so I was referred to an Urologist. So, my sick little buddy and I made an appointment to go and see the doctor.

As I arrived, the nurse at the reception desk gave me a choice of two doctors to see—my choice. Now perhaps I read into this more than I should, but I envisioned two guys. One very gentle doctor with well-manicured, petite fingers, and the other who looked like, sounded like, and had hands like Andre the Giant. I am sure that you remember Andre from the Princess Bride or from professional wrestling as I do, but I also remember pictures of his hands in an issue of Sports Illustrated. I remember that his hands were so big, he held a basketball in his hand that looked about the size of a softball. Another picture showed him holding a 12 ounce can of soda and his fingers were wrapped around the can and touched his thumb wrapped around the other side.

Now I had watched Let's Make a Deal enough times to know what happens if you choose the wrong curtain, but I did not have a whole studio audience screaming advice to me. I cannot divulge the name of the doctor I chose, but I will say that his name does include the root word of "high." I must not have been thinking clearly because I didn't even make the association of his name and the altitude needed for a real exact prostate size diagnosis. Actually, I thought that he must have "high" standards, or "high" sensitivity to the feelings of his patients. Believe it or not, and against all of my regular odds of fate and very bad luck, the doctor was very soft-spoken, and he really did have small, neatly manicured fingers. If you haven't seen Chevy Chase's movie classic, Fletch, then you can't fully comprehend the anxiety I felt as he asked me to drop my pants and bend over the examination table as he slapped on his rubber glove and applied a generous amount of lubricating jelly. Just as I was about to sing Moon River and "probe" with some questions of my own about the doctor's previous prison terms served, the exam was over and I survived it without any physical or mental scarring.

The reason why I mention this whole long story is that even though this was not a surgical procedure, it still deserves at least an honorable mention status in a man's writing of his medical memoirs. Now to the point of this alternate sign. My new intimate pal, the urologist, asked me if I had had trouble urinating including frequent trips to the potty to urinate, pushing in order to keep the flow going, and reset periods when you pee then rest, then pee and rest, pee and rest followed by the grand finale of dribbling at the end. You know what? All these years I have wondered why the old guys always go through this little ritual as they stand at the public urinal. It's not like I turn and look. That is just an unsaid rule—you never turn and look at the other guy standing next to you at the public urinal—even if you know them and even if they are family! You always keep your eyes on your own business while standing at a public urinal. But even looking straight ahead, you can still see through your peripheral vision that the old guy next to you is doing his best to eliminate down to the last drop. And now that I am older, I understand why. Anyway, I couldn't lie to the doctor. He was so kind and gentle and since we had now developed a special, intimate bond, and I knew that doctor-patient confidentiality lasted even beyond the grave, I answered in the affirmative to all three questions.

So, fellas, you know you are getting old when you dribble after draining, or as you may have guessed, I do have a nickname for it: Double Dribble. A sure sign of this is when you get those brand new, brightly colored gym shorts or leisure wear for you really old guys, and after you pee, you have to go to the hot air hand dryers (I hate those damn things for drying hands after washing! I understand the cost savings and the tree-saving concept, but I just hate standing there rubbing my hands together under the blower for what seems like an eternity—especially since I had to leave the opening night Clint Eastwood movie right at the climax because I have an enlarged prostate and I pee all the time. Only now as I am older, I realize that the creator of the hand air dryer whom I have wanted to give a prostate check personally only using his machine as a probing device, had the dribble disease too! So, he invented the air hand dryer to dry hands and to dry the wet spot right in front of your shorts—you know, the spot that is much darker and wetter than the rest of the shorts. The key to drying the spot is that you have to get to the dryer quickly so that no one sees this most embarrassing stain, and then you need to line up directly in front of the blower and rub your hands together just outside of the air flow to fake everyone out that you are in fact drying your hands while allowing for the air stream to get to the stain and dry it out so that even though it is still there, it now is the same color as your new shorts and you can quickly return to the movie!)

The thing that you need to be vigilant for with your new shorts is what I call, "Ring Around The Pee Pee." This is the yellow outlined water spot that shows up on the front of your shorts that means it is time for a good session in the washing machine. If you don't detect it, you will notice that while walking by females, they will point at the stain and look disgusted. Although this experience can be quite humiliating, you must remember that they are reacting to the stain, and not to your personal anatomy. It is much better to be found out by another guy—especially if he is older. He will just walk by you, cup his hand over his mouth toward your ear point downward with his other hand and say, "Hey, Dude—Double Dribble!" In either case, you find something to carry in front of you— even if you are forced to cross your hands in front of your soiled shorts—until you can get to that damn hand drier and do some quick rudimentary laundry with hand soap and water. Either that, or else you learn to carry a backup pair in your car for a quick change.

Chapter 2
The Two "Cystas," Pilonidal and Blood

Now I realize that the topic of cysts is a very sensitive one and so I cover this topic as one who has been very fortunate up to this point. However, I have had to face the waiting for results of biopsies, and I know what that waiting period feels like. I am not going to waste time here by discussing those little visits with the physician's assistant when he burned off some moles and growths. Those are trivial matters that are just a very normal part of getting older and are not worth mentioning here. With that said, I would like to talk about my experience with cysts to sprinkle this sometimes very hard dish to swallow with a bit of sweet humor. My first cyst (and I will admit that it did occur a little sooner than my 40th birthday so forgive me for fudging a bit, but I feel that it is an important part of my medical history, so I am including it at this point) hit me fast and hard. It started out to be what I thought was a big zit on my neck. The difference between this and a pimple was that pimples go away—even the tough repeaters and mirror shooters (sorry). This one seemed to grow even with the aggressive treatment that most zits receive. Finally, after about a month, I realized that this anthill was not going away and if left untreated, would look like one of those ant skyscrapers in the African bush! So, I made an appointment to see my good old primary physician who in turn referred me to an internal surgeon. This surgeon happened to be a friend of mine, and although I wasn't too concerned, I did know that one of his specialties was the treating of cancer patients. Our appointment was set very quickly, and I went to see him for an office visit. He took one look at the cyst and had me put on a gown right then and there so that he could remove it right on the spot. He deadened the area and then cut into my neck. I didn't feel any pain when he cut the cyst out, but I did see a splatter of blood shoot over the top of my head and I felt the warmth of the blood trickle down my neck and back. As he cut, he kept on asking me why I did not come in any sooner. I tried to explain that it came on so quick and I kept thinking that it would just go away, but it never did. I also told him that it had only been about five weeks since the thing showed up. Since we were friends, I kept on waiting for him to give me some warm and fuzzy words of comfort. But all I got was, "Why did you wait so long to come in and see me?"

After he finished cutting, gouging and stitching, he told me that this cyst, or I am pretty sure that at this point he used the "T" word (tumor), was one of two types. He said that if it were one type of tumor, I was fi ne and there would be no further need for treatment. Then he continued that if it were the other type or bad tumor, things "weren't good" and he would need to cut out some more tissue. Then he asked again why it took me so long to come and see him. I really wanted to tell him to stop asking me that, but I was a bit too scared to do so. Then I asked him how much more tissue he would have to remove. He told me that if it was the bad kind, he would have to cut down deep into my neck and shoulder and remove all the surrounding tissue and then treat the area to make sure that he got it all and that it would not come back. At this point, I really didn't have much more to say. Once again, I felt like suggesting to him that he should work on his bedside manner a bit, but I didn't. He told me that he would call with the results of the biopsy as soon as they came in. I left the office with about 15 stitches, a large bandage on my neck, and carrying a larger load of anxiety over having to wait for the results.

For the next several days, all I could do is wait and worry. I kept wondering if I should have gone in sooner and if it would have made a difference. And, I kept thinking about a bulldozer scooping buckets full of tissue out of my shoulder and what the big hole would look like. Fortunately for me, the call was all good news; the tumor was benign. In fact, the doctor explained to me that the tumor was known as a blood tumor that is caused by blood generating skin tissue growth. This type of cyst is fairly common and completely non-cancerous. Boy was I relieved and very, very fortunate! A big load had literally been lifted off of my shoulders.

The story surrounding my second cyst was quite bizarre. It all started when I noticed my underwear beginning to get wet—right in the middle of the top of my crack. Upon further investigation, I realized that there was a clear fluid coming out of my crack area, but not from my rectal cavity. I know that this sounds a bit gross to you but before you get too excited, just imagine for a moment how I felt about this whole event! I was worried that I would leave a puddle behind in the chair I was sitting in. And interestingly enough, my fluid flow fluctuated from time to time. I really can relate to how females feel when they face that time of the month when they experience changes in flow. I honestly contemplated purchasing some pads or something and I found myself wondering whether I should buy minis or maxis or just what I should buy. This was rather disturbing to me and frankly, it was sort of a threat to my manhood in a way. After a while, my condition got worse and my flow at times became heavy. I couldn't really figure out what was going on! All I knew was that the skin at the top of my crack area would get irritated from time to time, resulting in a release of slightly infected fluids.

Finally, I went to my primary care provider and he took a quick look and decided to refer me to a general surgeon. I showed up to the appointment a bit embarrassed, but anxious to get my leak plugged. Upon examining me after the good old "drop your drawers and bend over" command, the doctor quickly found the problem and told me to pull my pants back up. He told me that I had what is referred to as a pilonidal cyst, and that it could be easily corrected with a minor surgical procedure. He went on to educate me further as to the fissure's origin. Apparently, when babies are first born, one of the last areas of development is the closure of your butt crack (sorry, but I cannot remember the doctor's correct medical terminology that he must have used at the time). As the crack closes, sometimes it can overlap so that skin closes over skin. Now this does not become a problem until puberty when hair begins to grow. And (sorry) since butt hair really doesn't start to flourish like the Great Plains of the Midwest in the springtime until middle age, the problem doesn't flare up until later in life when hair starts to grow underneath this flap of skin. When this happens, and the area gets agitated from long periods of sitting, like at work for example, then a hole opens up and the fluids start to flow. The doctor said that this condition was quite common in men at this age. The way he explained it to me made a lot of sense, but I had never heard of it before. I guess that this condition isn't something commonly spoke of around the water cooler at work, or at the local fitness club. But then again, who would have the nerve to admit to something like this and voluntarily bring the subject up— unless of course you had just finished up with a meeting at work and everyone stood up to return to their desks and you were the only one standing there with a big wet mark on the back of your Dockers and someone yells out, "Hey Jim, did you just pee in your pants, or is it just a bad case of diarrhea?"

So, in order to fi x this, the doctor has to re-slice the crack and then partially stitch it back and then let the rest of the opened area close by itself the way it was supposed to close in the first place. And, he had to make sure that both sides were correct so that there were no more overlap containing hidden hairs underneath the surface. We scheduled the day of the procedure and it was a success. The ironic part of the healing process however, was that in order for this to re-heal properly, the doctor had to keep part of the flap open so that it would heal on its own. And, to make sure that there was no infection, he placed a drainage tube in the open area that came out around my backside to a drainage bulb that was safety pinned to my shirt in front so that I could empty the draining fluids periodically. For the next several weeks, I had this open area that really could not be bandaged that well—think about it and I'm sure you will get it—and I had to keep it clean and dry and drained of any fluids. It ended up being the month from hell! Finally, over a period of time, it did heal and fortunately for me, no hairs have sprouted up since.

Chapter 3

The Knees: Snap, Crackle, Pop, or Klunk

As I begin to discuss my knee situation, I must refer back to my physical characteristics and my past physical activity that play a key role in my continuing knee problems. First, I am 6'5" tall, and I weigh from 275 to 295 depending on what I ate for breakfast and on my ability to have good BM's on any particular day. Besides that, I participated in football as a defensive tackle, and in basketball as a post player throughout my middle school and high school days. And I continued to play basketball and racquetball for many years after graduating from high school. And when I began teaching high school, I was a defensive line coach for about 8 years. So, you could say that my knees received quite a pounding throughout my life.

My first significant knee injury occurred in my junior year in high school. I had twisted it, hyper-extended it, bruised it, and knocked it around quite a bit prior to that time, but one day while playing basketball, I planted my left foot, pivoted off of that foot, and spun around to take a shot. The problem was that my whole body twisted around for the shot, but my lower left leg at the knee stayed in the same place. This caused what you might call something bad to happen to my knee as evidenced by a loud popping noise that I both heard and felt as I fell to the ground in a considerable amount of pain. I must mention that this occurred in the spring of 1974. I must also remind you that during this period of time, knee surgery technological advancement had not progressed much since the dark ages. Arthroscopic surgery had not been invented yet, nor had Dr. Brown yet invented his back to the future time traveling DeLorean either. This meant that I had to deal with the current medical practice of treating knee injuries at that time.

The first doctor I went to was the local orthopedic surgeon in Boise Idaho where I was residing at the time. Now I am not bagging on Idaho as I love this beautiful state and I have great memories of growing up there. However, I do not believe that this particular doctor's methods were founded upon "leading edge technology." I remember going to see him with my mom. So, when my name was called, she went with me back into the examination room. Once the doctor came in and introductions were made, he asked me to describe what exactly had happened in the best detail that I could remember. So, I told him how I twisted the knee and I even tried to show him the direction my knee twisted and the angle at which it twisted and then I told him that as this occurred, I distinctly felt and heard a popping noise. As I explained what happened, he listened with attentiveness and as I described to him the noise my knee made, he stopped me and asked me if I was sure that it sounded like a "pop." I said that I was quite sure that it did in fact make a popping noise. And then, he asked me a question that I will never forget—one that made me not only question his medical competence, but one that when asked, my mom and I looked at each other in bewilderment and with all the strength we could muster due to respect for the medical profession, we held back a very strong impulse to crack

HEALTH, HUMOR, AND A HOLE IN THE WALL

up in laughter which we had to hold in until we left his office when as soon as we exited the building, we both laughed until tears were streaming down our faces and we had to sit in the car a while before mom was in the proper state of mind to drive home. His question was — and I hope that after that build up you are not disappointed that it isn't funnier except you really had to be there — "Now did your knee actually make a pop noise, or which noise did it actually make?" "Did it sound like a snap, crackle, pop, or klunk?" At first I thought he was joking. So I responded that I was pretty sure that it was a popping noise. He reiterated that it was very important for me to do my best to remember the exact noise that my knee made. At this point of the consultation, I was now confused, for after he questioned me several times as to the actual sound my knee made, I wasn't so sure anymore that it didn't make a "pop" noise at all. In fact, I was sort of leaning towards the "snap" or perhaps the "klunk" noise. So, after we went back and forth a few more times in this very intriguing Q and A period, he finally told me that he felt it was probably a torn meniscus and to just keep on playing basketball and participating in my other physical activities. In doing so the likelihood would greatly increase that it would ultimately tear all the way at which time I would for sure know that it was time for surgery no matter what sound it ended up making.

My mom and I left quite baffled by what the doctor had just said, yet highly entertained at the questions that the doctor had posed to us. Now as I look back on the incident, I wonder if the doctor didn't have an obsession for Rice Krispies and that his snap crackle and pop comment wasn't in fact rooted in some sort of sick attraction he had toward the three little Rice Krispy guys. The only problem with that theory of course is where the "klunk" came from. Maybe he researched the Hollywood try-outs for the commercial and there was a real hunk of a cartoon character named "Klunk" that didn't make the final cut for the commercial because he didn't really blend in with the other three. Maybe he was a bit too hairy or muscular and so he showed up the other three and made them look like sissy krispy guys or something. Perhaps we'll never know—especially now that I am quite certain that this doctor has kicked the bucket by now. (I wonder what specific sound he made as his foot struck the bucket! Was it a...)

Just a quick side note here: I love my mom very much. She is no longer with me, but her life and example will always be a great example to me. And, I am grateful for being born with her wit and her sense of humor. She had a favorite joke about my knee, which she was able to tell often as I dealt with the various injuries over the years. Whenever I would say that my knee hurt, she would always ask, "Which knee? Your left knee, your right knee, or your weinee?" Now I know that this joke is pretty corny, and you might roll your eyes, but just think—this joke came from my mother asking me this question while I was in my high school years. With that in mind, you have to admit that my mom was pretty cool!

The next step we took in fixing my knee was to get a referral to an orthopedic surgeon at the University of Utah Medical Center. My brother's wife's cousin (no joke) worked in that hospital, and somehow, we got in to see him. He did a great job in fixing my knee although it was anything but arthroscopic surgery! When he was finished, there was a scar all the way across my knee about seven or eight inches long, and I wore a full-leg splint for six weeks so that it could heal. I will not dwell on this surgery very long because it took place when I was in high school, but it does deserve mentioning as it did factor in to my knee problems of middle age.

After I got married and began my various careers, I continued to participate in football and basketball—both as a player and as
a high school coach. Now this participation consisted of playing on teams in church and city league teams as well as in pick-up games at local gyms. These games although are played for fun, can get pretty physical. And if you have played, you know what I am talking about. Some guys think that they are Kobe or Kareem, or Barkley, or LeBron, and their game tactics and behavior can sometimes get out of hand! They think that

they still have it and their minds tell them that they do. But their bodies and their reflexes, are just a bit off. This is due to the fact that their bodies are getting older, their reflexes aren't quite what they used to be, and they have gained about 40 pounds since their high school super star years! So their game is a bit rusty, their tempers are out of hand, and they place blame or call fouls on others to cover up for their faltering physical prowess! You who are now so called "hackers" or if you play with "hackers," you know exactly what I am talking about.

With my continued physical activity, my knees took a pounding. I can also say that further damage was done to my knees because I wasn't real smart when I chose my work out routines. Now days, we have a choice of a variety of low-impact exercise equipment to use to stay in shape. Also, I enjoyed going jogging and so with my large frame, I now realize that jogging just wasn't a very smart thing to do and it caused a lot of wear and tear on my already banged up knees from playing defensive tackle for eight years and almost playing more in college had I decided not to hang up the old cleats. Enough with the nostalgia. I will finish this chapter on knees by saying that I have had two surgeries on each knee over the last 15 years. These surgeries are basically to go in and trim off the little tares and "clean out" all the arthritic fibrous tissue that builds up over time. The irony is that my knee that required such a major surgery in high school, is now my "good knee!" Go figure! I am sure that one day in the not-too-distant future, I will qualify for a double knee replacement surgery. But for now, I am happy to go in every four or five years for a good old spring cleaning.

Chapter 4

The Double Hernia, Balls in a Vice Grip, Bowel-Imprisoned Air Pockets, or The Great Migration

I am not even going to discuss my first hernia surgery, as it did not take—whatever that means. I will just move right on to the second of my two hernia surgeries—the double whammy! To set the stage for this story, I must go way back in time to the days of young adolescent male physicals for sports participation. This experience introduced me to the concept that we could actually have a hernia. The doctor's procedure—and guys I am quite confident that all of you have had several—to check for hernia was completely humiliating and quite disturbing! I will skip the specifics on the procedure as guys will never forget and ladies most likely have heard the story before. I will however tell you that the very first time that a doctor puts on a rubber glove and tells you to drop your shorts, you are quite baffled. Then, as he sticks his two fingers up inside your little compartment and continues to push upward until you can almost taste latex in your mouth (before the days of scented rubber that some dentists use now when the taste could be a bit more like grape or bubble gum), he commands you to turn your head and cough! Now besides the fact that it seems the fi end's fingers are in your throat, thus blocking your esophagus from the capacity to even cough at all, and that you are standing on your very tip toes and without knowing it you have assumed a very difficult stance that is only achieved by ballerinas and boys having physicals, you desperately exhale much the same way that a king crabber gasps as he accidentally falls overboard into the icy waters of the Bering Sea! And, no matter how hard you try, this gasping refl ex is the only frail attempt at a cough that you can muster! But the relentless doctor presses on and commands you to cough again and again, and somewhere along the line, one of your rasping exhales is barely enough to count as finally, the fingers are lowered and your little buddies shudder with absolute relief. The result is that those twins are so traumatized, that they stay in hiding way up there for several weeks before they decide to come back down and join the party.

One side note is that a buddy of mine—also there for his first physical—came out of the exam room to where we were all lined up like pirates to the gallows with the most interesting facial expression I had ever seen. He appeared to be nervous, yet relieved; laughing, yet crying; animated, yet full of anxiety. As he came toward me, I could tell that he wanted to tell me something yet he was embarrassed to say it in front of the other guys. So I asked someone to save my place in line as we found a more secluded spot for him to confess his deed.

Now like Dragnet, what I am about to tell you is true. I will not ever divulge the name of my friend in order to protect the innocent. It seems that my friend was in so much shock as the doctor stuck his fingers into my friend's sack, and commanded my friend to cough, he turned his head and summoned all his strength and willpower and urinated in the doctor's hand! As we get together now, we still have a good laugh about his experience. The irony is that he is now a practicing doctor—and that is no lie!

With that personal background established, I will move on to my double hernia surgery. After the first go-round, I already knew the symptoms for lower hernia. For those who are not familiar to the symptoms, I need to make you aware of them so that you have fair warning. After all, how would you feel if everyone in your Florida neighborhood was notified of an impending level five hurricane while you were in the bathroom doing your business with the fan on, only to step outside to be swept away to Kansas by galle-force winds?

The symptoms of a lower hernia are very obvious. First and without any tact whatsoever, I will say that your balls feel like they are in a vice and Satan with his teethy, sinister smile spins the jaws of the clamp ever inward while jabbing the engorged imprisoned duo with his pitchfork. Next, when you cough, sneeze, pass gas, or take a BM, it feels like your balls just accelerated into the lead position of the Indy 500—outside of the race car and totally exposed to wind, debris, and big, hard-shelled bugs—with big fangs, stingers and pinchers. The third and only other symptom that you need to know—as if the first two are not enough—Is this: When you are standing up for any extended period of time. Your testes (sorry for my continued references to this delicate part of the male anatomy but it is what it is) feel like they are expanding, stretching, and elongating like starting a slinky at the top of the escape stairwell of the Empire State Building.

Now you would think that the repair of this type of condition would be quite relieving—well, in the famous words of The Great Karnak to Ed McMahon, "You are so wrong bar rag breath!" The end of the surgery was only the beginning of my problems. After surgically implanting and interweaving a NASA-grade fibrous mesh into both sides of my lower abdomen, they closed me up with stitches and covered them with cloth tape. Then, they sent me home to recover. They did warn me that I could have some post-surgery air pockets in my upper abdomen that I needed to pass as they could feel "uncomfortable." They counseled me that if this condition did arise, to walk it off and allow the air to "dissipate." The surgery was claimed a double success and I was sent home with a wheel chair ride to the family van.

For most people, this would be the happy ending to a nice story. But for me, this was the beginning of a saga worse than the original Nightmare on Elm Street through the tenth sequel. I don't mean to be disrespectful to religious epics, but looking back on the experience is kinda like the children of Israel being told by Moses that he was going to set them free and then once they escaped, they had to endure crossing the Red Sea, standing in what must have been a never-ending line to get a drink of water flowing out of a rock, only manna from heaven to eat— without toppings, and the hurling of the tablets of stone containing the ten commandments with the ensuing wrath of God, just because they made a few statues to "dress up" their wilderness home!

As I arrived home and crawled out of the van, I realized that I couldn't walk without a great deal of pain. I also noticed— here it goes again—that my testicles had enlarged a bit. "A bit" translates into something like two basketballs encased in a water balloon. They hurt all the time. Next, I noticed that I had some trapped, high-abdomen air pockets as foretold. So, as instructed, I tried to walk them off and dissipate the gas. I took a pain pill, got up off the couch, and began my trek. After about five steps, I realized that my pilgrimage to the Gods of entrapped air was in vain. Continuing on was pointless. I couldn't walk any further nor could I fart, so I went to plan B. I crawled back inside to the family room and knelt on the floor. I recalled in my state of agony and frustration that air bubbles trapped in liquid travel upward. With this sudden revelation, I continued my supplication, calling upon heavenly intervention as I assumed the proverbial angle in which my face was in the carpet and my rectal opening was pointing skyward. At that moment and as if on cue, we received a divine visitor (literally)—the head shepherd of our local religious flock. He came by with his wife to see how I was doing.

Little did he realize that the very foundation of his core of religious fundamentals would be put to the task. After exchanging pleasantries amidst the unusual circumstances, as I had not changed my position, my inspirational leader asked if there was anything he could do for me. At this very moment of my desperation, I don't think that he could fathom what he was actually asking. I wanted to respond by requesting that he relieve the pressure by popping the basketballs and squeezing the crap—I mean air out of me. But since his wife was present, I just asked him for any ideas to relieve the symptoms of bloating and constipation. What came next made me realize how pathetically old I was becoming as our conversation for the next half hour centered around all the different varieties and procedures of a topic that I had not ever tackled to this point in my life—that of enemas!

And so with a smile on their faces and with their faith intact, they bid farewell as my wife got back in the van and headed off to the drug store to buy the desperately sought after remedy, while I anxiously awaited the divine gem with baited butt breath, remaining in my position of supplication.

What happened next is rather vague in my conscious awareness. Back to my psychology background, perhaps I am suffering from post-traumatic stress disorder, but I will do my best to finish the story so as not to disappoint you.

My wife returned with various boxes full of bags, hoses and nozzles, and we used ALL OF THEM—at least twice! And yet, after all of the vigorous rectal bingeing and purging, the air pockets remained. Ironically, to this day I have yet to read about another case of rectal bulimia.

Now armed with a renewed determination and with a spotlessly clean colon that could support the controlled environment needed to manufacture computer board capacitors (and with the needed newly remodeled expanded square footage to do so), I went to plan C, since Plan B was self-annihilation. Plan C consisted of dragging myself outside to our backyard basketball court and setting baby step goals. My first goal was to walk until I released some air. That goal ended up with the same amount of success as the guy who set his sights on earning his first million dollars by purchasing one lottery ticket a week.

After that goal failed in the first two limps, I decided that I would hobble one length of the court before resting—about 50 feet. With the determination of "The Little Engine Who Could," I completed the first lap. As I crossed the finish line and began my resting period in a doubled over position and in the thrill of victory, I felt a long familiar, yet somewhat distant to the present, urge to release some gas. With great anticipatory relief, I squeezed off an encouraging yet somewhat disappointing tweeter sounding very similar to the ending note of Dumb and Dumber's Harry at the end of his episode on Lauren Holly's plugged-up toilet after purging the Turbo Lax. This moment of false hope led to despair as the next two laps resulted in similar very small victories. I finally gave in to the realization that the air would escape when it was ready to do so just as the Alien creature would burst out of it's victim's exploding chest only after the full gestation period had been completed.

So, I came inside, popped another couple of pain pills, and went to bed. And then, somewhere in the night, not dissimilar to an innocent child's eager anticipation of Santa's magical trip down the chimney with all those long-awaited treasures reserved solely for the most special of the bestest girls and boys in the universe, the event caught up with me and I found fulfillment. The air flowed like the dews of heaven as my lines purged like the Alaskan pipeline after an environmental impact study on the habitat of the rare Alaskan critter—the sphincticus analcolonoscupus.

And now, was the journey complete and have we reached the end of the story? Not hardly my friends! Not even close! That's like saying that we have no need for another Batman sequels! Like cake without ice cream, Like bread without butter, Like George without Gracie, Like—well you get the idea.

In the famous words of Paul Harvey, "Here's the rest of the story."

Let's get back to the cloth tape that was used to cover my stitches. At this point I should interject that through this experience I gained a great personal insight. I would be exaggerating if my epiphany were compared to the discoveries of a round earth or gravity or even pizza—I found out that I am allergic to cloth tape. Now that's bad enough as it is but this is me talking here, so of course, there's more.

To add further enlightenment to this story, I need to go back in time about 25 years to when I had just entered high school. My oldest brother had just returned from a long stay in Taiwan. My other brother and I asked him if he would bring us home something cool when he returned. We weren't expecting much as our elder brother was quite cheap, but he actually brought us home two very special gifts. The first, for which we sent him money and which cost half of what we paid, were a couple of real neat swords with hand-carved sheathes covered in all different types of ancient oriental royalty depicting great ninja battles of historical significance, but in our ignorance, we knew not what. The second gift, which was really the first and only gift he really brought us since we paid for the swords, was a doozie! He brought us some sort of jungle rot dreaded gamboo jock rot! That's right. During his stay in Taiwan, our brother had contracted some strain of fungus on his scrotum that made the black plague of the dark ages look like a small blemish on the huge rump of an elephant. This stuff predated the Big Bang Theory, The Ice Age, The Great Continental Shift, and Global Warming. It is more resilient than the cockroach, more destructive than a nuclear bomb, faster than a speeding bullet, more powerful than a locomotive, and able to leap whole continents in a single bound. You get the idea. This was very, very bad stuff. It could have been passed on to us by a satanic, sold-her-soul-to-Satan Hooker from hell, but since we were completely virgin territory at that tender age, It was passed on quite innocently (on our part) to our genitals, separately of course, through the use of a common bath towel that hung so threateningly yet ever so innocently on the towel rack next to the shower like a Venus Flytrap lazily smiling in the morning dew awaiting the two juvenile fl ies that were nearby playing catch with a piece of dog turd. Through the generosity of our eldest brother, he wanted to share his Taiwan experience with us in a more intimate fashion, so he made sure that he used the same shower towel that we used. Then, he completely and thoroughly wiped his tainted genitals with our towels after his shower. As a result, we know for a fact that he was a repeated offender, as we both immediately contracted the fiery disease that quickly progressed into advanced stages.

My brothers and I all played high school football. We had experienced the usual athlete's foot where the skin burns, itches, cracks and even bleeds. But comparing that to this rash is like comparing my financial portfolio with that of Bill Gates and saying that my net worth is about equal to his (Remember, I am a school teacher.). Back in those days, we didn't have a lot of alternatives to treat severe rashes—you know—the bleeding kind. So, once our ninja warrior rashes (that kept pace with each other) got to the point where no over the counter medications helped and our crotches and scrotums looked like Mount Saint Helens during and immediately after the blast, we decided to take drastic action. So, we gave each other a big pep talk to psyche ourselves up including the alternative of becoming Eunuchs, who really don't have a place in modern civilization, and we got a big, high-speed box fan and a jumbo-sized bottle of rubbing alcohol. (I always wondered why the name included the word "rubbing" until this experience occurred.) Now I am absolutely convinced that we must have shared a very similar skin-melting condition with the creator of rubbing alcohol who also had to use it for serious rubbing applications), and we headed for our bedroom. Then, one at a time with the other keeping watch to make sure that our parents didn't come in and see the carnage, we would go into the bedroom, drop our drawers, sit in front of the fan set on high speed and apply or rub on if you will the alcohol in abundance to all of the afflicted areas and surrounding healthy tissue—or what was left of it—to stop the spread and to burn the rash out. The fan would confuse the pain receptors on our skin into thinking that the drying alcohol was actually providing a soothing sensation in some absurd neurological networking malfunction. This kind of brain functioning mess up is kind of like turning the key of your car in the ignition and instead of starting the engine, your car disintegrates into a mushroom cloud. Fortunately, the human body has other fight or flight mechanisms when faced with a situation of sheer terror and intense agony that in some weird, dropping acid sort of way— hurts so good. But, we knew better because the floodgates of our tear ducts flowed so freely that we immediately became severely dehydrated and of course, our private parts began to bleed.

Truly, I am amazed that ten years after this episode, I was able to have children with my wife. After this ordeal, you might think me suspicious of the mail man or milk man or grocery boy as possible fathers of our children, but I trust my wife completely, and my children look like me and share some of my somewhat unique characteristics, and oh yeh, I did have a DNA test done on each child just to be sure—just kidding!

Now, where was I—oh I remember now, back to the hernia surgery and the cloth first aid tape.

I found out that I was very allergic to first aid tape of the cloth kind, and I soon found out that the ensuing rash made my Taiwan Testicle Terror episode seem very juvenile, much the same way that watching Barney on TV is a bit different than renting "Texas Chainsaw Massacre." Even though this analogy could be quite accurate if you do ever have the misfortune of contracting this rash as a result of selling your soul to the devil, signing the contract in your own blood, and then telling Satan afterwards that you made a mistake and you were wondering if you could just put all the past behind you and part your separate ways as friends. If this were to happen to you, you would certainly—as I did—consider using a chainsaw to destroy the beast (another reference to the devil)—the rash I mean.

This rash reminded me of a brush fi re rushing downhill with the assistance of galle-force, fi re-breathing winds through the now lifeless, brittle skeletal remains of a lush hillside that was once a wavy, emerald green sea full of our fellow earth friends that provided life-supporting oxygen. After the demonic rash dragon breathed his last breath, the only microscopic particles left behind after the incineration that could be identified by a CSI team was a final exhale equal to a crusty old cowboy who after smoking four packs of non-filtered cigarettes a day for fifty years, let out a final breath that did not cloud the distorted glass pained window of the local saloon on which he expired with a moist fog, but instead left a thin, crusty, white dusting of old tobacco breath ash.

You might think that this analogy is greatly exaggerated to add humor to the story, but unless you were one of the rare few who witnessed the event, you would be the same as someone who read about nuclear testing in the desert during the 50's, as opposed to one of the special military clearance personnel that were at the sight and had their shoes blown off of their feet even when standing in a so-called protected area.

Anyway, the rash started to spread southward toward the peninsula and the adjacent two small islands. I was reminded of the destructive path that the stampeding herd of buffalo left behind after the big hunt in "Dances With Wolves." Loaded with knowledge from a previous rash experience (refer back to the Taiwan Testicle Terror if you dare), I reacted quicker this time. I got out our much newer and quieter yet same CFM air-flowing box fan, a bottle of generic but equally potent rubbing alcohol, and went to my room to reenact the biological skin war. Then, in order to protect the children under the age of 18 in our household, as this particular material was certainly not suited for their psychological well-being, I locked the door. As I turned on the fan, lined up and sat down on the bed while dropping my drawers, I said a prayer and opened the bottle of alcohol—rubbing alcohol that is. Taking a deep breath while mouthing the word "amen," I poured a bunch in my hand and applied the liquid super generously.

What happened next was as unexpected as a fi reman laying down what he thought to be a blast of fi re-quenching water, only to see the blaze explode to life as the water had somehow been replaced with a very volatile rocket fuel solution. As I applied the alcohol, the burning sensation intensified, unsubdued by the flame-retardant imposter. And even though the blood did flow, the rash began to accelerate in velocity like a Swiss Alp avalanche. So, I applied some first aid crème of some kind and called the hernia doctor. Recognizing the desperation in my high-pitched screaming and pleading, the doctor fi t me right in. I put a towel on my car seat and headed down to his office.

After fidgeting around on the uncomfortable waiting room chair for what seemed to be an eternity, during which time I was getting stares from women tightly grasping their small children = probably because of the bizarre movements and uncontrolled twitching that my hands, arms, and legs were gyrating, I was called into the examining room to await the doctor. The nurse showed some concern as she took my blood pressure, body temperature, and pulse. My vitals must have been in the red zone due to my high state of trauma. To relieve her concerns, I explained that I had a post-op hernia rash that was causing some discomfort. She nodded her head, scratched down a few notes and exited quickly. I don't think she had any desire to do any sort of pre-exam. Soon, the doctor entered and inquired as to the reason for my unscheduled return visit. As I told him of my post-op condition, he said, "Okay, let's take a look-see. Go ahead and pull down your pants." At this point I am confident that the doctor was not prepared for, nor did he have the extensive medical training in infectious diseases, or working in a war zone triage, or autopsy work for the coroner for what he was about to see. For, as I dropped my pants, the escaping toxic heat wave took his breath away, singed off his eyebrow hair, and blew off his classic combover. I had the sudden urge to offer him a Tootsie-Pop and say, "Remember Who Loves You Baby!" But I didn't. He let out a little gasp and an expletive and said, "Wow!" "I have never seen anything like this in my medical career. I am going to have to consult my partners and call a specialist in infections." Then he asked, "Do you mind if my colleagues come in and take a look?" At this point in my life, I have very little pride left, let alone conceit, and so I responded, "Hey, why don't we bring in all of the nursing staff and we can have a party!" We had a good laugh, he called in his buddy, and he got me some prescription strength hydrocortisone cream. After a very long two weeks, the soothing balm of Giliad took effect and the fi re subsided. And that, my friends (After all the intimate experiences I have shared with you, I can call you my friend even if you would rather not ever be associated with me or even be in the same building with me.), is the rest of the story!

Chapter 5

IVs, Transfusions, Catheters, and Jumbo Wipes

This story really begins over two years ago when I had my back fused. My back saga is a story of it's own, but the prolonged recovery of that surgery leads into this fascinating and true story. Part of my recovery process included pain medication. I am not proud of that fact, nor am I proud to say that I was popping pills sort of like Kobayashi eats hot dogs. I even had to stop watching the TV show House because his addiction made even me feel guilty. I'm not going to change directions and get all tender and soft on you in this chapter, I just want you to know that I was hooked. The crazy part is that I did not fully understand until I went to a pain management doctor that once you start taking those damn things, they run your life. Your schedule is all centered around your next little hit. More than ever before, I can now relate to the guy who sells his soul to the devil for one more hit. I must confess that I did not get far when I prayed for more "relief." Apparently, God knew that what I was asking for is like a pyromaniac asking for some gasoline and matches and promising not to burn anything! I must admit that calling Satan did cross my mind, but fortunately, the welfare of my eternal soul pricked my conscience and kicked me in the butt with some common sense.

This revelation was aided by my pain management doctor, who weaned me off the junk. He informed me that the more you take opiates for pain, the more your own brain's ability to distinguish back pain from the nerve's cry for more drugs diminishes. In other words, Your back may be completely fi ne, but your nervous system and the brain are so addicted to the meds, that your nerves send the same signal to your brain that scream back pain, when actually they are screaming for more drugs! I learned from "painful experience" that I would probably feel these errant messages for the next six months, until my brain had a chance to replenish my own natural pain-blocking neurotransmitters. So while maintaining my full schedule, I was motivated to get clean in 21 days and I did so. For any of you who may be in this situation, I have some advice. Get off the pills. At some point, they build up a resistance and they just don't work anymore, yet you are compelled to take more and more. And, once you have made the decision to stop with the assistance of a doctor, there are painless ways to step down off of the pills and finally purge your system of these death feeders. The key to your success depends on the motivation and determination that you have once you make the decision. There is absolutely no feeling like getting your life back!

Okay, sorry for the soap box, but if I can help anyone out there get unhooked, then that's the least I can do for those who helped me.

The human body is an amazing machine. Normally, it functions on an extremely efficient level. Another little tidbit of knowledge I learned the hard way is to listen to your body when it speaks to you. What I mean is, usually when there is something wrong, your body will send you warning signals. While I was on pain meds, I had hot flashes at night, I felt nausea, I had severe pain centered right at the point of my sternum, and all I could eat were crackers and a little soup. Going through these symptoms was a scary time for me because I thought that all of these symptoms were related to drug withdrawals, when in fact my body was sending me frequent and intense warning signals, flashing like a highway patrolman in your rearview mirror at night! I further thought that if I did get off the junk, I would have to go to rehab and pull a Ray Charles or Johnny Cash gig in the local padded cell hotel. (By the way, sometimes rehab includes checking yourself in to a reputable facility in order to properly monitor your health and help ou deal with issues in your life that may cause you to crave the stuff. So if you need to check yourself in—do it now for yourself and for all who love you!)

The crazy thing about all these so called "withdrawals" was that they were actually DEFCON 5 alarms sounding off inside my body that I had a major health problem, but they were disguised by my ignorant ASS-umption that they were all withdrawal related. So, when I was completely free from the junk, I really got sick! I went to the doctor a few times, was misdiagnosed as having acid reflux, and sent on my way with a few prescription strength antacids. Fortunately, the doctor did order up some blood work and so a few days after my visit, and with continued pains centered in my sternum area and still awaiting my referral to a gastro-intestinal specialist, I went and had the lab work done. (At this point I will say that I am grateful to have insurance, but HMO's getting referrals approved could probably be compared to staying up to witness Haley's Comet streaking across the night sky when it had just passed by the earth last week!)

When the blood work was interpreted by my doctor, he gave me a phone call that went something like this, "Well, your blood is all out of whack and since you are experiencing chest pains, I don't think that you are having a heart attack, but I think that you should go to the Emergency room right now just in case." I must admit that getting this message from my doctor is like being invited to a toga party yet after you get there, you realize that that you are attending a regional KKK meeting, and you're the only African American in the room and all of the exits are blocked by big guys named Billy-Bob, and Super-Tanker, And Spud-Nuts, and the total number of teeth in the room besides yours which are still intact, equals one and a half.

I was scared, and a sense of panic came over me unlike I had ever encountered. The doctor did say that the symptoms could also point to gall stones and that I should get an ultra sound for my gall bladder while they are looking at my heart. At the time of the call, I was in my classroom. After hanging up, I got up out of my chair and noticed a deep gouge in my chair. Upon further examination and removal of fabric and foam cushioning out of the rump area of my jeans, I realized that the gouge was in fact, the legendary sphincter bite-marks that I had only heard about but did not think could actually occur! Boy, did I underestimate the power of the rectum! Come showtime, that thing can really do some amazing contortions, which I will describe later on in the chapter. Immediately after the bite mark episode, I got someone to cover my class and headed for the emergency room.

As I arrived at the ER and waded through the triage of the sick and wounded, I was very happy to see that the physician on call at the emergency ward was a friend of mine. You'd think that I was on a first name basis with all doctors within a 100-mile radius of my home, but I did associate with this one outside the medical setting. He put me at the top of the list and called me in to the exam room. I told him that I was either having a heart attack or else I was having a gall bladder problem, or I had one of those little aliens growing inside my chest as I referred to earlier. He checked my vitals, drew some blood (Are we still blood-letting in this day and age of modern medicine?), and determined that my heart was fi ne. He then decided to get out the sonogram machine and either check my gall bladder or check for the reptilian embryo—he could do both at the same time as they are located in the same general area. Fortunately, he did not find an alien, but he did inform me that I had gall stones and that I needed to be checked in to the hospital to get them removed. So, they stuck in an IV, put me on a gurney, and rolled me into the elevator and up to my new room awaiting the surgeon's visit. I did not have my own private room. I did have four or five roommates. I guess that this was sort of like a holding cell until the jury could confirm my gall bladder's guilty verdict. Looking back on it now with the enlightenment of "The Bucket List," I am certain that Jack Nicholson owned this hospital as well as the one in the movie.

Before I continue, I must say that I do not drink or smoke or use drugs—except for the ones authorized and certified by the medical field. And by the way, I am not blaming my doctors for my dependency problem. I understand that a genetic predisposition to addictions runs in my good old family tree, so I know that if I indulge once, I will probably return to the good old vomit as a dog doeth. So, I try to stay away from the vomitus substances.

Because I was experiencing some pain and I was under the care of physicians galore, when the nurse asked me if I wanted something for pain, I started salivating like Pavlov's dogs would have had they been served heroin instead of dog food after hearing the bell. I was no less excited than if she were a server at The Chart House reading off the choices of surf and turf! So wrapped up in the analogy, my veins were crying out for the liquid equivalent of prime rib, lobster, and the baked Alaska, so I asked, "Well, what are my choices?" She then proceeded down the list. The first stop was morphine. I drooled. I asked, "What else? as if the variety of catches of the day had just come into the harbor in a large freighter from salt water heaven. The waitress continued. "We also have dilauded." The corners of my mouth twitched in anticipation as the new word was now firmly engrained into my list of must remember vocabulary words. "Tell me about it." I swallowed. She responded that it was an alternative type of pain medication that was about seven times more potent than morphine. I choked. Mustering up all of my self-control not to just scream out "Yes! Yes!! YES!!!" (Sorry but the anticipation was intense!), I responded, "I think I'll try that one." "The dilauded?" She asked. "Yes, the dilauded" I responded. I quivered.

As I said before, I do not smoke and I do not drink. In fact, I don't gamble anymore because I can't stop trying to earn back the long gone twenty I blew moments before which had been sucked down the swiftly flowing refuse of cheap buffet smudged wads of soul-selling cash that flowed into the cash pipeline that fuels Sin City. What happened when the nurse injected the liquid platinum into my IV and as the fluid cursed through my longing veins, is as difficult to explain as how it must feel. I imagine that this moment of intense pleasure could be best compared to— you know what? This time I will let you fill in your very own fantasy of extreme and intense pleasure imaginable—that's what it was like. As I sat back and felt the warmth flow through my shuddering bones, I visualized rubbing my chapped, frigid fingers in front of a freshly stoked wood-burning stove after a long day of survival tests with Bear Grills on the bitter cold ice fields of Greenland. Now I have never actually been to Greenland, but just the mere thought of being exposed to this type of extreme experience made my scrotum tighten. By the way, this primitive genital reflex is actually a flight or flight defense mechanism that has been etched into our evolutionary human genetic code since the first Cro-Magnon man figured out, as he was watching his friend become the daily special of the neighborhood saber-toothed tiger, that he had better get the dinosaur poop out of there! So guys—galls I am not sure what your equivalent sensation could possibly be—wherever you are and whatever you are doing, when this reflex occurs—RUN like hell!

I do not remember all of the details that occurred over the next several hours, but I do remember asking the nurse with a façade expression of euphorically disguised discomfort how long before my next hit—I mean medicinal injection. She told me that I could have more every four hours. I looked what appeared to be miles away down my arm to the watch which was spinning and glowing and morphing before my eyes much as in looking through a kaleidoscope of sensory overload. I think I know what Timothy Leary meant when he said that while high on a hallucinogenic drug, you can actually taste color. This particular sensory feast was more satisfying than Thanksgiving dinner! Anyway, I focused all my weakened sensory faculties to visualize the mirage glimmering on my watch face. I etched the time into the stone tablets of my mind. I don't remember much about that first day, but I do remember that I was renewed with the living waters flowing from the fountain of youth and psychedelic wonders every four hours to the nanosecond!

Unfortunately, I have one more very vivid recollection of day one that even a crack-meth cocktail could not have erased. Throughout the evening of day one, and as my veins were being transfused with the embalming fluid of concentrated ecstasy, I must have mentioned to the nurse that I had a difficult time urinating. The nurse mistakenly interpreted the fact that my chart showed that I have an enlarged prostate, which could possibly be the cause of a urinary tract blockage. I cannot dispute the enlarged prostate, but I can say that I could still pee, even though I had to push a bit and the result was always a bit of dribbling. I tried to tell him that urinating all the fluids and medications and antibiotics that were being pumped into my IV by the turbo-charged NASA fuel injection system, was like urinating Hershey's syrup. He either got irritated at my language or he was simply following orders from his supervisor, the princess of darkness, because immediately after our conversation, he brought in a demonic device which if I remember correctly, even has a big sticker with Satan's smiling face right on the front of the package. This device, created from the very bowels of Hades itself, is better known as a catheter. I need to emphasize at this point that my catheter insertor was a male nurse. I guess they thought that I would be more relaxed with a male nurse. This ended up being a very overestimated assumption. After all, who would you rather be handling such a delicate piece of equipment? If you were going to cut a priceless gem, would you use an expert jeweler, or would you go down to the nearest construction site and get the jack hammer guy named Joe and tell him to cut away? Never-the-less, the male nurse came in to do the procedure.

From a non-medical point of view, the catheter is an absolutely horrible device with an even horribler (not misspelled since it is worse than more horrible) idea behind it. Assembly and insertion includes some lubricant (not long-lasting), a tube about four or five feet long, a big bag, and an injection syringe. I will now explain the purpose of each. First came the lubricant. This is used at the insertion end of the tube to allow for the tube to go in easier. In concept, that may be a good idea. However, in reality there is no such thing as an easy insertion—as I was about to find out. Think of a freight train passing through a pup tent and you can get the idea. The male nurse told me that I might experience some discomfort. Unfortunately, that part of my body had never experienced this type of procedure before, and so it was not at all prepared for what was about to happen. Now that it has happened to me on four separate occasions, my anatomical part is very prepared. In fact, now when I even see a clear plastic tube, he (Do you mind if I refer to it as he?) goes into sudden and immediate hiding, the same as a turtle under attack by a vicious canine.

As the nurse was lubing the tube, he mentioned that during insertion, I should take deep breaths—sort of like Lamaze breathing. He notified me that it was time to start my deep breathing. The result of my reaction while he inserted the foreign device was very similar to my wife's response when I told her to breathe during the birth of our first child, only she was more polite than I was. After all, in my wife's case of giving birth, I was her husband. In this case, I really had no relationship with this male nurse although now I feel a weird sense of bonding due to the intimacy of his actions. My wife screamed at me that her pains of giving birth were somehow all my fault, that she hated me, and I smelled and to get out of there—right before she began to ask forgiveness and beg for my return. This behavior repeated itself until she gave birth. In the case of the catheter insertion, I did not give birth, but my nervous system burst with an explosion of nerve cell transmissions as I screamed things at the nurse that now I almost regret. I know that I commented on his lineage (family), perhaps even his parents and their marital status. All I know is that it was extremely painful and although my memory of the event is very fragmented, I believe I recall that I pleaded for a double dose of dilaudid. Then, he secured the tube to the bag and got out the syringe. I couldn't imagine what use a syringe could possibly have and so I inquired. He informed me that in order to ensure that the tube did not fall out, he would inject some air into a small fitting on the tube to create an air bubble inside me to secure the tube in place. Have you ever regretted asking a question that you really had no desire for an answer— or at least a truthful one?

After this, I remember trying to relax and lay back in bed with my tube and bag, my IV, and with the clear fluids that I was only allowed to eat. Speaking of which, I still to this day cannot figure out how a hospital can screw up the recipe for chicken broth. Now let's see, oh yeah, here is the recipe. Get a big pan, add broth and simmer until it is hot! Or how about the recipe for Jell-O? Boil water and add Jell-O, then stir, cool and serve. Where in there does it mention that you add some horse poop? Is the hospital chef on furlough from the local medieval asylum? I was sick, hungry, peeing in a bag, and all I could eat was Mr. Ed's turd soup!

I was starting to feel a bit queasy at this point, and I really wasn't very hungry anyway, and so I lay down to try to get some sleep. You would think that at the very least, I could get some sleep in a hospital. Well, I had further obstacles to overcome. First of all, every time I began to doze off, someone came in to prick or probe. I also found out real quickly that if the length of the tube to my bag was anywhere near the side of the bed, it would get bumped by staff or visitors walking by my bed. The bumping or tapping of the tube—no matter how slight—would send a reverberating shock wave down the tube to the entry point, just as an 8.5 earthquake on the Richter Scale would send shock waves violently down the length of the fault line. Once the calamity took place a few times, I realized that I had to take precautionary measures. The turtle was getting very nervous and scared. And so, I carefully took the tube from the point of entry and placed it running down the middle of the bed, protected between my legs, until it crossed the lowest barrier—my ankles—and found its way to the bag hanging on a hook alongside the foot of my bed.

I will say that my wife gave me great comfort during what ended up being a nine-day ordeal. She was always there, day and night, to help me out or just keep me company. She would get me little juices or help clean me up or make my bed. She even bought an eggshell foam pad and brought it to me and made my bed with the pad on top of the mattress and under the sheet so that I would be more comfortable. There is nothing that made me feel better than just knowing she was always there for me—and I love her even more for it. With that being said, I was completely at her mercy as I was quite immobile. And, I am not sure if I became paranoid or not, but to this day, I think that somehow, she took advantage of my helplessness and very subtly got even with me for those few times which she accused me of not showing her the kindness and sensitivity that I should as her husband. She will deny this, but I believe that she would tap my tube every once in a while just to let me know who was really the boss. When she arrived in the morning and leaned over to kiss me, she would tap the tube. When she made the bed, she tapped the tube. When she placed a drink on my tray, she tapped the tube. And every time she tapped the tube, I would fl inch and express my concern. She would always apologize but I am convinced that when she tapped, the sides of her mouth curved upward in an ever so slight twitching grin. To this day, she denies it, but I think that she tapped on purpose.

At this point, and with the intoxicating medications I was receiving, you would think that I was in relative comfort. How wrong you are, hospital cafeteria chef's surprise breath! For, I really was having a very difficult time releasing the Hershey's syrup, even though it now had a pipeline direct to the reservoir. In fact, I felt like there was a system back up of some kind building up similar to the upper abdomen air pockets of my double hernia surgery only in liquid form. Being quite baffed at this frustrating predicament, I visually followed the tube downstream and noticed that the stream bed looked something like the one where the outlaws are crossing the treacherous, wind-blown desert and all that is left of a once flowing stream is a layer of flaky, warped tiles of dried dirt. And, as I looked into the bag, I was horrified to see that all that the only substance that had made it that far was reddish in color. Now I am no doctor, but even when I drink red punch and eat strawberry crunchy cereal covered in strawberry milk, I have never peed red, so I pushed the call button on my bed. That's another thing about hospitals. What's up with the call button? No matter how you loop it, tie it in a knot, coil up the cord and place it by your ear to watch TV or to call the nurse, it ends up on the floor and out of reach without straining the tube along with the body part attached to the other side of the tube! Why can't they just put a button on the controls of the bed, or give you a small wireless radio, or just give you a can on some string hanging from the ceiling. Sometimes—and I'll explain in further detail later—you need that call butt within a quick hand's reach.

The nurse at the other end of the call button informed me that she would send my nurse right down. The nurse this time was female—thank goodness—and she was very sweet, and petite and cute and soft spoken. I am so glad that it wasn't Helga the Horrible with big, callused hands whose only previous employment took place in war-torn Eastern Europe by performing a primitive technique of hacking off limbs! How could I have known that such a sweet person could deliver the news I was about to receive. In her cute little voice with a slight Asian accent, she looked at the bag and with delicate concern, she told me that the catheter had been inserted incorrectly and it would have to be removed and reinserted. It might just as well have been Satan in the room with all his hosts of hell telling me to come on in and join the campfire! The turtle jerked and immediately went into hyper-hibernation. But, the pain was awful—even without any tapping—and so as she reassured me that she would be gentle and that if done right, it really wouldn't hurt as bad as last time, and so I agreed. She retrieved a new kit and prepared to make the switch. She then took out a syringe and inserted it into the fitting and sucked out the air bubble. I felt a slight twinge of relief. Inside the shell, the turtle opened one eye and peeked to see what was going on. The sweet little caretaker of my manhood told me to take a deep breath and then exhale as she removed the tube. I took a big gulp of air and tried to disassociate myself from my body. I was wishing for an out of body experience, but all I could settle for was a full-body shiver. As she began to remove the tube, I exhaled. I don't think that I said anything to offend her, but since she was so pleasant, I'm quite confident that I could have reacted like a drunken sailor and she still would have said, "Now that wasn't so bad, was it?" I'm quite confident that I left some permanent teeth marks in my tongue and in my underwear and breathed a great sigh of relief! The turtle dared to move ever so slightly. Then, came the bad news. She needed to redo the procedure with a new catheter, as she was quite certain that my bladder was in need of relieving. This is like receiving the death sentence, having it carried out through the method of the electric chair, then the chair malfunctions, giving out only a near-death, but still conscious jolt of electricity, resulting in the legal technicality that your sentence was not completed and so you have to get hooked up to old sparky for one more go at it!

So, I started my Lamaze method of breathing as she greased the next tube. I was trying to hyperventilate and pass out. It didn't work. I asked her to make it quick. I felt like I was facing a fi ring squad and the guys were passing the time playing Go Fish. She inserted the tube as I bit a hole in my lip and sucked in blood and saliva. My mouth sure throbbed but so did the little turtle who by now was about to go to the SPCA for animal cruelty. While the intense pain was passing much like a kidney stone passes, the nurse said, "All finished," as if she were just polishing off a donut. I wiped the sweat off my face, the blood and drool off my chin, and the poop out of my shorts (as best I could), tucked the tube oh so gently into the valley between my legs, and laid back on my pillow. I think I can relate to amputees of the late 1800's—no sedative, crude equipment, and phantom limb pain. Although I felt like I still had a limb and it hurt like hell, the battered and bruised little guy had long since vanished.

Day two found me visiting with my surgeon. When she first came into the room, she looked at my name on the chart with a puzzled look on her face. As she realized who I was, she asked me if I wasn't supposed to see her in her office the next day. I told her that since my wonderful HMO (Doesn't that sound like some kind of negative oxy-moron—Wonderful HMO? How can you use those terms together?) took so long to get me an appointment with her because I kept on getting bumped from my appointments due to her constant visits to patients who had already smartly checked themselves into the hospital, I had to wait too long and my doctor told me to just go to the hospital and she would show up there quicker. So, I ended up bumping some other poor sucker who was patiently waiting their delaying turn to see the surgeon. She checked me out, looked at my chart and the sonogram report, and told me that she would be performing my surgery and removing my gall bladder. She said that the attacks that I had experienced over the past several years were actually my gall bladder passing stones. I sure wish that I would have known that say two years ago! She scheduled my surgery in two days. She then informed me that before the surgery, I had to have a small procedure called an ERCP to have a stint placed in the tube running from my gall bladder to my intestine to make sure that there were no stones in that tube as they could cause problems or a blockage later. She said that it was a minor procedure that lasted about 45 minutes and that I was scheduled to have it done by a gastro-intestinal specialist the following morning. She mentioned his name and said that he is the only doctor in my area that does this procedure. The nurses reassured me that he was "very good at what he does." That seemed comforting. In reality, that is like being reassured by an unfamiliar doctor making a routine house call that ends up being Jack the Ripper.

An ERCP is perhaps one of the most disturbing and certainly the very worst part of having your gall bladder removed. The morning of the event started out the same as usual—Jell-O, broth, and juice, followed by a dessert of dilauded. Then, my nurse told me that I would be going in to have the procedure done sometime during day three. As I sat around waiting, I started to get a bit antsy. In fact, the anxiety of waiting brought on a new symptom that I had never before experienced. I later learned that this freaky thing I was experiencing was called "anxious leg syndrome." All I know is that all of a sudden, my legs started wiggling and getting this feeling that a million ants were crawling all over my legs. As if they had a mind of their own, they started to twitch and jump and wiggle, and the more I tried to control it, like a very bad cough, the worse it got. Finally, I had to jump up out of bed and take a walk. The nurse asked me where I was going and all I told her was that my legs were freaking out and I had to get out of bed and walk or run or jump out the window or something. I just had to get out of the room and be doing something with my legs, and I had to do it right now! Because my vitals were not real stable at this time, my nurse was concerned about my taking a walk. But, I had to get out of there. What I wanted to do was tear out my IV and catheter— air bubble included and take off bare-bottom completely exposed down the hallway wearing nothing but that stupid gown that would have been short even in mini-skirt standards. By the way, you know that a gown is too short when your belly button shows below your gown hemline. Instead, the nurse allowed me to take a brief walk around the room and sit back down while she gave me something to calm my twitching nerves. Unless you have experienced anxious leg syndrome, you cannot relate to what I am saying here. I almost asked for them to strap me down like a meth addict, but I focused real hard and finally got to where my legs returned from their record paced marathon and rejoined me in bed. Then, I waited and waited until around 8:00pm, when I was finally called down to the surgery level for the procedure. Not that I would have eaten anyway, but I was refused liquids all day and by that time, I was hungry and very thirsty. Munching on a very meager cup of ice chips during the day does not satisfy thirst just as much sucking on a mouthful of snow quenches your thirst while climbing Mount Everest. My tongue was now the size of a football and my legs were convulsing in seizure-like form, but I was ready to get this thing over with.

They brought me a wheel chair and offered to place my catheter bag on a little hook. I instinctively grabbed the bag and said that I could carry it myself. The instinct was brought on by an idea that popped into my mind that the hook was loose and that while they were whisking me down the hallway, the bag fell and was run over by the wheel chair causing the tube to become taut and the air bubble inside my abdomen located somewhere between my bladder and the turtle to be tested as to its engineered specifications to not explode outward, thus releasing the bubble and the tube to be jolted out, leaving only the burst remains of what was once my manhood. The gurney guy (These are the nice guys that work in the hospital who have the sole job description of wheeling people around in wheel chairs and hospital beds.) wheeled me down to the butchering block—I mean the surgery room and I was met there by a nurse who explained to me the procedure that was about to take place. She was as calm as a summer morning and as stone cold sober as Hannibal Lector taking the stand, as she described this simple procedure as Hannie (as he was called by his closest friends) would recount his dining experience with the Psyche Ward prison warden. In that little procedural description, the nurse informed me of several key bits of info that caused my rectum to grab onto the gurney. First, she told me that I would be awake during the procedure. To this day, I am not quite sure why this is necessary except that perhaps it reduces hospital costs. So, instead of keeping me awake, I don't understand why they wouldn't just knock me out with medication and then cover the cost by raising the "hospital price" of a generic Tylenol to $100 per tablet instead of the going discounted rate of $50.

Never the less, I was to be awake. She did say that I would be receiving a "Twilight" sedative that would make it so that I would not be consciously alert and aware of what was going on—Yeah, right, little Miss Lector! She also casually mentioned that I would be lying on my side and there would be a mouthpiece to hold the tubes going down into my stomach and intestine to where the stint was to be placed — "Whoa! Back up there little angel of darkness! You say what? There are tubes going where?" All of these exclamations entered my mind as she was talking, but the shock caused my brain to freeze the nerve signals to my mouth and vocal chords to express them out loud. With tears swelling in my eyes and a twitching mouth, I affirmed that I had received the message—not that I understood, let alone agreed with what she was saying. Since I already had an IV, she told me that she was going to give me something to relax me and put me in a "twilight" state. She might just as well been the star of the book made movie Twilight leaning over to inject my veins with her serum-injecting fangs. I did inform her that I am a large adult male—about 6'5" weighing about 285 pounds at the time, and that I had been on pain meds for previous medical conditions (yet to be explored in this writing), and that I had built up quite a tolerance for meds over the years so she should be generous.

I felt like I was asking Ebeneezer Scrooge for a donation to the poor house—before the three ghostly visitors after midnight. She nodded her head while scheming on how she was about to rid the world of it's surplus population. She took the route of the IV instead and told me that I would soon be very relaxed and consciously floating off to my happy place. If my happy place were hellfire and damnation, and I was playing tag with Freddie Kruger and Jack the Ripper, then she was right.

She laid me down on my side and asked me to open my mouth as wide as I could. To the best of my recollection, the mouthpiece appeared to be just like Dr. Lector's headgear. It stretched my lips to the point of ripping flesh. It had about a one-inch diameter hole in the center for the tubes down my throat. Once the apparatus was in place and the involuntary swallowing reflexes began, and without the ability to communicate except with gasps, wide eyes, uncontrollable rectal spasms evidenced by some very high pitched farts since the sphincter had gone into lockdown, and my middle finger, the nurse informed me that there would be five tubes down my throat continuing into the stomach and on into the small intestine. These tubes were made of a sort of metal fl ex hose I assume because they were going to pass through some pretty strong fluids—although the table where my anus was situated had now collected some of those fluids that should make the trip down the gastro-intestinal highway a little less cloudy. In the sheer panic that ensued, I remember that Dr. Satan, Son of Darkness (at least that is the name and title that I remember him announcing as he entered accompanied by a host of ghastly demons and assorted phantasms of the underworld), came in with a smile and introduced himself briefly as he announced that we needed to begin as long as I was ready. Little did I realize that my state was actually the Twilight Zone and he was Rod Serling! Rod, I mean Satan asked the nurse if I was ready and if I had received enough of the sedative. She nodded in the affirmative as I mustered up all my strength and squeezed off a referee whistle fart I hoped would sound something like "No way in hell am I ready!" Apparently, Lucifer doesn't speak fart and so he began. I was wide-awake as he approached me with the hoses. Did I say tubes before? Well, these suckers were hoses—all five of them. They felt like searing-hot pitchforks.

I remember that as he slid the hoses back and forth to get to
the right place, and fortunately one of the hoses was attached
to a small camera although it felt like the size of a camera you
see in television studios, I gagged when he moved the pipes
forward and I wretched when he backed them up. This went
on for quite some time, perhaps due to a foggy lens. I know
that the nurse saw and heard my silent screams, gurgling, tears
and gurgling rectal reverberations because on three different
occasions, she asked the horned red guy disguised in a lab coat
if she should give me some more sedative. Each time she
asked, I nodded my head violently and made some kind of
noise that I hoped she would interpret as a yes. Finally, after
the fourth injection of what must have been a placebo, I finally
either responded or passed out. Either way, I was alert for 20
minutes of the half hour procedure and I will never forget the
sheer terror that I felt as I endured what must feel like an
impalement from Count Vladimr Dragulia, or whatever
Dracula's name was while still mortal.

Finally as the terror ended, they then wheeled me back to
my room and I crawled back into bed to be rewarded with
some more broth, Jell-O, and herbal tea that I left untouched
as I am sure that it would have just dribbled down my neck
anyway. For the time being, the No Vacancy sign was flashing
at the entrance of my mouth and the entryway was closed for
major repairs. Fortunately, I could still be served my newly
discovered favorite meal—the dilauded injection. By now I was
hoping it was being served Las Vegas buffet style with
unlimited refills. I wanted to binge until I purged and then feast
again. Unfortunately, I could only pass through the line once,
and I couldn't have any seconds—not even visit the dessert bar
full of lard-frosting pastries—for another four hours.

I refer to day three as the green mile. This was the day of my final hours before the gall bladder surgery was to take place early the next morning. I remember waking up to a feeling of nausea. I was confident that this was brought on by my system's desire to purge itself of the previous day's debris, or it was my body telling me that I had exceeded the limit of consuming that dog-diarrhea clear-liquid diet I had been on for over 48 hours. So, when I realized that vomiting was inevitable, I carefully grabbed the yellow bag with one hand, my IV cart with my other hand, and shuffled over to the bathroom. Now if you are like me, I absolutely hate throwing up. I try to sleep, or at least lay perfectly still for the regurge urge to pass, or I just sit there and just moan and try to will myself to get better. As I do so, I focus all my willpower and visualize passing the acidic fluids on through my digestive system and blowing them out the other side. One of the worst things I have ever had to do in my life was to stick my finger down my throat to induce vomiting. I think that hanging myself would actually be less traumatic. It would also be a quick, sure-fi re cure for nausea and I would be in denial if I did not admit that the thought had never crossed my mind. It takes all of my will-power and complete mind control to force my clammy, trembling hand to my mouth, then extend my frozen finger outward and place it on the back of my tongue. But there are times when the cramps and nausea become more intense than the fear of sticking my finger down my throat, at which time I am able to muster enough courage to do the deed and self-purge.

Sorry for the visual, but if you have been through this, you know exactly what I went through. However, in this case, I knew that the flow was coming, and coming fast, so I assumed the position of worshipping the porcelain gods. The flood gates opened and they flowed freely. In fact, I was amazed at how easy the process was. No finger, no retching, no convulsing. It was like I was singing only the music was not so melodic, just a rushing of waters and a splashdown, like a waterfall if you have a real good imagination. If only all vomiting was that easy. The song was real short—only one verse—and so I got my bag and my IV cart and returned to my bed. The process went so well that I felt as though I had been blessed by some divine intervention as a merciful act of recompense for the purgatorial ordeal I had passed through the previous day. There I was, feeling better and even considering a bite of Jell-O when the urge to purge returned, and return it did with a vengeance!

Have you ever had one of those times when you knew that you were going to purge and you had absolutely no control over the contortions and convulsions that your body suddenly commenced without any warning whatsoever—not even a little twinge or gag reflex? Well, one of those times suddenly hit me while lying there recuperating from the first session. In a desperate panic, I got up, grabbed the bag and IV cart, and ran to the little shared bathroom. Fortunately, none of the other patients were occupying the beckoning fixture. Otherwise, I would have hurled all over some innocent victim of what could be referred to as a fl y by spewage. As I entered the room, I placed my bag on the door handle and dropped to my knees as if to pray. However, as I tried to supplicate for the sparing of my life, The capacity for speech was incapacitated by a gaping gag best compared to that of a great white shark or a vicious anaconda as they dislocate their jaw in order to consume their fresh catch of the day. The other horrific side of the ordeal was that once the gagging commenced, there was a huge time lapse until the meager fluids of unknown origin finally surfaced from the very depths of my bowels—like some translucent sea creatures finding their way to the surface from the deepest, uncharted oceanic trenches. Fortunately for me, just at the brink of blacking out due to oxygen deprivation, the greenish goo made its way out and plopped into its new porcelain home. To this day, and I have purged many times before, I have never retched to the point of turning my insides into my outsides with the end result of having hemorrhoidal tissue dangling from my lips! The event was so traumatic, that all I could do when I was finally finished was to just sit there on the floor with my head leaning against the toilet bowl. The coolness of the ceramic fixture brought some relief as I tried to control the trembling and twitching until I could gather enough strength to move. After a cooling off period, I gathered my composure, tucked the hemorrhoidal tissue back into my mouth and crawled back into bed.

This procedure reoccurred several times during the morning to the point of considering making a call to Doctor Kivorkian to pay me a visit to assist me with alleviating my condition. I finally figured out that I was having a negative reaction to the precious dilauded that caused the awful side effects. I know now with complete clarity how a heroin addict feels when they get so violently sick from coming down off of their last hit. I was not hooked yet, but I was facing a dilemma. I could either continue with the good stuff and deal with the violent side effects, or else I could settle for something a little less potent— like morphine. It was kind of like settling for the meat loaf when the steak and lobster were the same price. However, since the steak and lobster symbolically had just announced a recall for botulism, I wisely settled for the meat loaf. It still tasted real good and satisfied my neuronal craving.

Day four began as expected. A nurse came in to awaken me with a big stack of forms to sign away any possible procedural accidents, life-threatening side effects or death or any other conceivable negative effects as a result of the surgery. I was surprised at how many potential risks were involved if I was fortunate enough to survive the procedure. After I autographed every page of the surgical liability and full disclosure packet, I asked for one more pain injection for my newly acquired writing cramps and carpal tunnel syndrome. I wonder how many attorneys and the number of malpractice suits it had taken to write this what would have been a best seller, with over a million copies in circulation, if it were a suspense novel. After the autograph ceremony was completed, the wheel chair guy came and got me and took me down to the operating room. The cool air and the pleasant music felt good. I laid down on the operating table and after a blanket was placed over my exposed lower trunk area—which by now I could really care less who saw what, where or when, the anesthesiologist gave me a little tour over her procedure that would later be billed by the minute. At this point, I was introduced to my all-star cast of support staff ending with a quick visit with my surgeon. (By the way, I need to do a little shout out to my surgeon. She was awesome! In fact, her dealing with my surgery and complications was so professional, when I went to visit her for my post-op checkup over a month later, I brought her flowers. She told me that had never happened to her before and she had our picture taken together with her holding the flowers.) Then, the anesthesiologist placed a mask over my nose and mouth and asked me to count backwards from ten to one. I think I got to about "te" when I lost all consciousness.

Those of you who have gone under general anesthetic for surgery, know what it is like when you begin to come out of it while in the recovery room. Some of what you go through definitely depends on how long you have been under while the surgery takes place, and what has been done to you while you are on the carving board—exposed like a Thanksgiving turkey waiting on the table with all the starving family members hovering anxiously around the feast waiting for grace to be said. I was under for about four hours. I vaguely remember opening my eyes but not sure whether or not I was awake or involved in some weird dream. I remember feeling a lot of pain and asking for more medication. I also remember that moving my head made my stomach churn with the rolling motion of rogue waves in the midst of a hurricane. I remember fighting off the urge to purge and fell in and out of consciousness over a period of about two hours. And no matter how hard I fought to stay awake, I did not have the capacity to control my level of alertness, my spinning head, my churning gut, and the pain in my abdomen, so I desired and welcomed the periods of sleep and I took full advantage of my waking moments to plead for more drugs.

After getting the green light from the recovery nurse and enjoying the post-surgery celebratory dining experience of a Styrofoam cup of ice chips to moisten my crusty Sahara Desert lips, the wheel chair guy, who doubled as the gurney guy brought me back to my room where I found myself the sole tenant, even though there were three other beds. And so there I lay in my bed with a flimsy curtain offering me a bit of privacy for I don't know what reason, since I was so warm that I lay there in bed dressed with my gown up to my neck, a damp washcloth on my forehead, and a dry washcloth covering what little private area I had left. My only other occupants besides my wife were the IV cart and the catheter bag, and a new friend, a drainage bulb and tube that exited my wound that collected bloody fluids still seeping from the wound. This bulb was about the size of a baseball, only oblong, and it was squeezable so that it created a suction to draw out the fluids. I still felt quite nauseated and I also had heartburn, so my meds were expanded to include an anti-nausea medication and a strong acid reducer. I also made sure that I got a hit of morphine every four hours to the second. My IV cart held bags of fluids that would be my source of food, vitamins, and a super dose of antibiotics over what ended up being the next five days. Other fluids would be added which I will get to in a little while.

While stabilizing in bed watching the news and being comforted by the mere presence of my wife sitting at my side, my surgeon came in to tell me how things went. As she described what she found when she went in, she was quite amazed. The reason why I had been so sick for so long was that my gall bladder had over 50 gall stones, it was black—meaning it was totally dead, and it had gangrene. And because it was gangrenous, there was some infection. It was the worst she had ever seen in all her hundreds of gall bladder surgeries. She almost had to cut me open all the way across my abdomen to remove it without it bursting, but she was able to secure it, isolate it, contain it, and remove it intact. She told me that it was a ticking time bomb that could have burst at any moment and if it had, I would be laying on a cold metal embalming table at the local morgue instead of in the hospital bed. But, in spite of it all, I was feeling quite well all things considered, and she asked me if I wanted to go home the next day if I continued to feel okay. She did say that the infection would have to be monitored and that she was hoping that by the next day, the blood would stop seeping out of the wound and into the tube. I told her that I would like to go home, but I wanted to stay until the bleeding stopped. Little did I know that the bleeding would continue for five days and require three blood transfusions of two pints each time. If you do the math, an average person holds about 14 pints of blood and I had to replace six of those over the course of the next five days.

I will interject right now a huge and sincere expression of thanks for all those out there who give blood. Whoever you are—you saved my life and I am indebted to you. Just don't show up at my house and expect to move in or anything. Just accept my sincere and literal heartfelt thanks.

I have to say in retrospect that this decision of mine, although the correct one, ended up like my taking a road trip up the coast. When at the point of falling asleep at the wheel, I pull into a small lodging facility named Hotel California—a place where you can check in, but never check out. Then by miraculous means, an escape was executed with a clean getaway back up the highway. And feeling relived that you survived a certain and undesirable death, you continue to drive on up the highway, and with great relief, you find a nice quaint little roadside inn with the unlit sign covered by trees. You get out of the car, stretch out your arms and stroll up to the office to check into your new beckoning sanctuary. Little do you know that the hidden sign reads "The Bates Motel!"

I firmly believe that part of the delay in my healing process was that I was not allowed to sleep. The desire and the dire need were there, but the opportunity showed its head on very rare occasions and for only a brief moment. Looking back, I would say that I had about the same chance of getting some sleep as I did having Pamela Anderson dropping in for a visit to see how I was doing and laying down next to me to give me some comfort by running her fingers through my greasy, stinky pillow hair and whispering words of comfort and encouragement into my ear— all within the presence of my wife sitting by the side of my bed reading People magazine and unaware of my visitor, thinking her an elderly nurse coming in to check my blood pressure. There I was, in bed and in my skimpy nightie with the lights down low. But every time I closed my eyes and started to drift off, someone was there to probe or prick or check my vitals, or someone would tap the catheter tube.

The next day after the surgery was quite uneventful. I found myself with very little to do, nothing that I wanted to eat—I mean drink as I was on clear fluids. So, I spent most of my time watching TV and meticulously and repeatedly lining up the catheter tube between my legs and trying to keep everyone off limits—except when the nurse came in to empty the bag and measure my urine output. I couldn't eat anything, I couldn't sleep, and I started to feel real sick. All I had to look forward to was the morphine and a little bit of apple juice that my wife snuck into me—which was the only thing that tasted good at that point. My vital signs started to go to hell, and I continued to seep blood at over a pint a day. As a result of the continued seepage, not all of the blood was making its way to the tube. Sometime that evening as I went to the bathroom to wash my face a little, I looked into the mirror and had a very frightful experience. You know in the movie when the minor part actress looks into the mirror while washing her face and all of a sudden, her face begins to stretch and melt off her skull and blood and brains come spewing out causing the mirror to shatter? Well, I had a similar experience except that the mirror remained intact. As I looked at the three small scars on my abdomen, I was horrified to see that a basketball sized, deep purplish bruise had formed on my side. The only difference between this startling visual experience and the one at the movies is that at some point, the movie is going to advance on to the next peaceful scene to set up the next seat jumping, scream-inducing, mask-disguised slasher, while my scene remained frozen on the crystal screen and I couldn't go and ask for a refund. This huge bruise actually looked worse than it sounds. It was so tender, that I had a hard time sitting up, let alone laying on either side. So, all I could do was lay on my back and gain a much greater sympathy for people who lay so long that they get bedsores. I had not developed any open sores at that point in my stay, but the stagnation was causing my backside to feel like Megatron had just knocked me through a brick wall!

The only good news at this point was that my condition was now upgraded to serious. I think that that is like getting a seating upgrade on an airplane from business class to the luggage compartment below. In this worsening state, I was moved to the next floor up and placed in a bed in a two bed, curtain partitioned smaller room in the PCU unit. This is the floor right below the ICU. I was hoping that I would not be getting that next level upgrade since there is only one more after that which is the morgue and that is just a tad bit chilly and permanent for my taste. I was now confined to the bed so that even if I wanted to go for a little stroll down the hallway and show off my hairy, sagging buttocks to a group of third grade students and their teachers singing and spreading cheer throughout the hallway—which I thought about doing just for some kind of entertainment besides the television's monotonous news and game shows—I had to stay in bed. And besides, there were no third graders around anyway, just a bunch of other middle-aged patients walking the hallways with their IV cart also showing off their hairy, sagging backsides as they tried to work out their post-op bowel movement that had now been log-jammed up for over three days. This move of mine to the next level of care upstairs was certainly no Hilton upgrade to a suite. My bed companion status—meaning guys in the same room in different beds and with different conditions, went from me being by myself in a four bedroom to me and a roommate in a two bed room. He was right on the other side of the totally non-soundproofed curtain.

The condition of the guy next to me was not good. Most of the time, he was on a humidifying mask to help him breathe, although from the sound of his coughing, I was surprised that he had any lung tissue left intact. And, if he wasn't coughing, his wife was gabbing in the most piercing, obnoxious tone that I felt like what a dog must go through when going through obedience training with the task master using a super high-frequency whistle in shaping appropriate behavior. On top of that, my roommate and I had to share the same TV. And, since my roommate was there first, he sort of had first dibs on the choice of channels. He stuck with the news and game shows. I hate watching the news and any other game shows besides The Price is Right—at least while Bob Barker was still there. If I wasn't listening to the TV, I would have to endure my roommate's neurotic wife who was constantly jabbering on for what seemed to be hours, as if her husband's healing was completely dependent upon the number of words she could squeak out per minute. And, she was only silenced by her husband's coughing up half a lung as he had pneumonia as well as a heart condition that caused his breathing to be labored and raspy and chunky.

Because of my sporadic vitals going crazy, I was given a little monitoring device that had five electrode wires that were attached by a very strong adhesive to the hairiest parts of my chest and abdomen. And due to my hairiness, the electrodes kept coming loose as recognized by the nurse running into my room thinking I had flatlined and preparing for a code blue (I have acquired such a medical lingo over the years!). And so, she would yank it off along with a clump of hair big enough to provide Telly Sevalas with a full toupee, and she would then stick another electrode on to a nearby patch of undisturbed hair. I have now become much more tolerant of environmental issues like destroying the rainforest and unregulated tree harvesting as I recall the symbolic similarities between my chest and the demolished rainforests. For when I was all finished, my chest and abdomen looked like the 40-year-old virgin—large patches of bare skin, void of any growth whatsoever.

At this point I will reveal that I am a religious person whose faith was about to face the supreme test of a lifetime which I will explain later. And since I am religious, I need to make a little confession. I admit that I was praying for some privacy so that I could get some sleep. Remember the old saying that you need to be careful for what you pray for because you just might get the answer in a very different form in which it was asked. Well my prayer was answered in two ways. First, my companion's condition started to deteriorate and he along with his wife were transferred to ICU. I really do hope that he got better and that he had a very temporary setback that divinely corrected itself once he was moved. The second act of divine intervention was that since I had not had any sleep for three days now, and when the nicest, sweetest, most soft-spoken petite nurse came on duty and came in to see how I was doing, I demanded that she remove the catheter so that I could get some sleep. I don't think that I was very polite and I kind of remember telling her that if she didn't remove it right now, I was going to yank it out—air bubble and all! She told me that it wasn't a good idea and that the resident physician who ordered it in the first place would have to approve the removal. I guess that this was one of those times when I needed to use my training in tough love. She was so nice, but I got tough. I didn't get physical or anything, and I knew that if I was rude, she would just leave, so I pulled out of my bag of tricks the one typically used by females on a highway patrol officer on the verge of issuing a ticket. So with all my energy, and focusing all of my emotions on the memory of Old Yeller and Where the Red Fern Grows, my eyes teared up as I pleaded for some relief so that I could sleep. And, the reality that I had not slept in three days teamed up with the moist eyes struck a chord in her angelic nobility and she agreed to remove the turtle-killing device from hell. Sorry but I still get all worked up about the demonic device.

And so with some deep-breathing techniques I had developed like a mom performing Lamaze to distract from the pain of her third delivery of an infant who was arriving about a month late, the nurse removed the catheter tube. To put it as delicately as possible, the ecstasy of the moment far exceeded anything I had encountered before. And although the turtle had been placed on the endangered species list, he had survived to propagate his species for another day—although I knew there was absolutely no possibility of any future baby turtles for this family. In fact, once we had four children, I told my wife that I had a dream that we had a fifth child, a boy. Now if you adhere to the Sigmund Freud theory of psychoanalysis, then you would agree with me that dreams have a very deep and significant meaning. So, as I described my dream to her in great detail and with great enthusiasm, I told my wife that it was a sign that we should have another baby and that he was waiting in heaven to be sent only to us. Her response was not quite what I expected. She told me without any hesitation in her voice whatsoever that I had her complete support and agreement to have another child — with one little important directive. If I were to have another child, it would have to be with another woman because she was through!

Now guys since our part in child bearing is so easy, the wife does really have final say on when and how many. And I would add my little take on having babies. If men were faced with the voluntarily allowing our body to get to the very gates of death being escorted by the guy in the black, hooded cape and his scythe, and once there, we would have to crap a watermelon, then mankind would go extinct! Men absolutely wimp-out when it comes to pain and we just wouldn't do it. Women on the other hand, not only go through this incredibly difficult biological metamorphosis in order to bring a precious life into this world, but after it is over and they have had time to recover, and they deal with this incredible challenge of working so diligently to get their figure back to where it was before the train wreck, many of them decide to go through the whole thing again! And for some, again and again and then again! That is why women are so special and why they truly are very different from men. And, that is one of the many reasons why we as men should hold women with such high regard, respect, and admiration.

But for me, I had just been given permission to go out and seek fertile soil elsewhere in which to plant my seed! I am still searching for my heaven-waiting son's new mother, and most of the candidates are way too young and gorgeous that make the reality of the union seem utterly laughable, and I know deep down in my heart that I would never cheat on my wife. I love her too much and she has learned to tolerate me and our four children are so awesome that I would never be so stupid as to jeopardize what I have when it is really just too good to be true.

Get out a tissue and let me get on with the story.

Finally, after three days of sleeplessness, the nurse turned out the light, shut the blinds, and I drifted off into a peaceful slumber. And, just as Pamela, the Hawaiian Tropic Swimsuit team, and all of Hefner's roommates entered into the hospital to pay me a heartfelt visit of tender comfort, my little angel of mercy caregiver entered the room and promptly woke me up sometime during the wee hours of night four. My beauty sleep and my beautiful guests were ripped away from me as I gained consciousness, and I realized that she was no angel at all, but a very wicked, wicked witch and her house had just fallen on me. For no sooner had I woken up, she informed me that the resident doctor, Der Fuhrer, had ordered her to replace the catheter immediately or I was to be shot for treason at dawn— or something to that effect. At the sound of this, the turtle almost leapt from his shell to seek out a new home in anything suitable—even an occupied bed pan. And so, my worst possible nightmare became a reality. She got out a new kit: lube, tube, and bag, and once again, I did my best to practice Lamaze breathing and all of the cuss words that came to mind, distracting me from the intense pain as once again the turtle was impaled. After the merciless act of violence that should be included in the Geneva Convention's chapter entitled "Improper and Unacceptable Practices of War Prisoner Treatment" was completed, my senses began to return. I laid back in bed making sure the new tube was securely in place down in the valley between my legs and centered down the middle of the bed.

Because of my mandatory confinement to the bed and feeling quite like the kid with the ankle transmitter in "Disturbia," I really didn't have a lot of options to keep myself busy. Little did I know that the transmitter, had I worn one, was about to go off like fi reworks on the fourth of July. I had been mandated by Adolf or one of her SS, that if I had to go to the bathroom, I was supposed to ring the call button and request a bedpan. I knew that I was quite safe because my fluids were all being taken care of and since I couldn't even eat (drink) the liquid diet daily special of herbal tea, consume, and Jell-O, and all I was sneaking into my system was the contraband apple juice that my wife was smuggling in, I knew that I would have no need for a bedpan. Once again, the Great Karnak would say, "How wrong you are, cesspool breath!" For I had failed to realize that all of the nutrients and medications and antibiotics and other substances that were being fed me through various bags, tubes and IV's when combined in the blood system, actually are bypassed by the liver and kidneys that put up a "No Trespassing" sign, forcing this newly formed band of criminals to find refuge in my intestinal tract. Even worse, my colon ratted them out, called out the cops, and now instinctually reacting to an evolutionary state of "fight or flight" mode, these hard-core criminals had nowhere else to go but be forced out in the open for the big showdown!

Because all of this criminal activity was perpetrated by key moles secretly working on the inside of the organization—or in this case—inside my bowels, even I was not privy to the impending massacre that was about to break out. Suddenly, and without any warning or even as much as a little tingle, I knew that I had to go number two. And what I realized with eyes enlarging to the size of those of Homer Simpson, my sphincter had seen the smoldering mob now gathering strength in numbers and pushing forward with ever increasing momentum, and suddenly and without any notice had immediately evacuated the area, leaving the floodgates of doom wide open. Apparently, my colon's call for help fell on deaf ears, or perhaps like the boy who cried wolf, the cops had shown up one too many of these movements before, and so I was left all alone to face pending doom.

I fumbled for the call button and with the only energy I had left as all reserves had been called out to hold off the intense rectal spasming, and with as much self-control that I could muster, for the first time in my life I asked if someone could bring me a bedpan. And as the nurse at the desk responded by telling me that she would be sending someone right down, I responded with the zeal of a William Wallace war cry, "She has about eight seconds—Go! Now!" I dropped the call button and focused all my will power on holding it in. I was actually hoping that my doubts on telekinesis would be overcome by my intense mental energies somehow holding back the floodgates of toxic refuse.

The nurse took nine seconds and the ability to move or in this case, hold off the movement of objects, failed.

My sphincter had betrayed me.

My nurse pleaded to the gods of super heroes for superman to fl y around the word and cause a reverse rotation to bring back the clock just for one second. There ARE NO SUCH THINGS as the gods of super heroes, and there IS NO Superman!

I know that my face looked like the kid that couldn't sleep on Christmas Eve and so he went downstairs and was just opening the last present under mom's immaculately decorated tree with all the presents neatly arranged around the tree apron, when dad came down the stairs after the cookies and milk and their eyes met. She was so nice and kind. (I would have quit right then and there! That is why there are more female than male nurses.) Her reassuring response was so comforting that my tears of humiliation dried up as she said, "That's alright, just let me know when you are finished, and we'll get you cleaned up." Fortunately for them, they had previously laid down some jumbo-sized pads on my bed which I was laying on; their maximum strength of absorption was to be tested far more than any paper towel or toilet paper commercial had gone before.

I normally don't get into details about poop, although I have heard guys brag about theirs and I have even heard that some idiots actually take pictures for display on the Internet, but I have no personal witness of this unsettling activity. However, in this case, I can go into a brief description because this stuff was not even biological! It was chemical! If Minute Lube could somehow bottle this stuff, a car would absolutely never need another oil change! The combination of stuff being pumped through my veins, mixed with a little bit of hospital contraband apple juice, flowed through me like ocean water gushing into Titanic. But the consistency and color of the fluids appeared to be more like anti-freeze than ocean water. I guess that this gives new meaning to the phrase: flushing out your old radiator fluids. There was absolutely nothing I could do about it but stick around and hope for a lifeboat or even just a flotation device.

The nurse waited what I imagined must have been the longest, most painstaking ten minutes of her life, when she entered and stood by the side my bed as a pillar of strength and politely asked if I were finished. I looked at her with a child-like grin as if I was caught in the act of lifting a cookie out of the cookie jar after being told not to take any cookies, and I thought for a moment while taking a mental evaluation of how far along I had advanced in the purging process. Then, realizing that my bowels were still quite unstable and that even though the volcano had already erupted, the bubbling, churning molten goop was in the process of erupting several more times, I sheepishly grinned and shook my head no. She smiled and said to just let her know when I was finished. This sequence of events repeated themselves two or three more times in the space of about a half an hour when I finally was able to respond in the affirmative that my work was complete. If this situation would have been an art class assignment of exploring with color and texture, then I had just painted a masterpiece! The nurse called up the reserves and they left the room for a moment. When they returned, they were fully equipped for the task at hand. They looked like a HAZMAT team just entering the scene at the disaster at Three Mile Island. The devastation was comparable. They brought out the biggest bag of magnum jumbo butt wipes I had ever seen! These things were big enough to handle any industrial sized job. If only they were around for the Valdez oil spill, the oil slick would have been contained so much quicker and the clean up a snap! Anyway, the team cleaned me up as if I were Baby Huey, changed my gown, and sheets, and filled up an entire red 30-gallon trash can marked "Hazardous Waste." They also disposed of their no-longer-sanitary suits, gloves and masks into the receptacle that would soon be dumped somewhere in the middle of the desert or depths of the ocean.

By this point in my life, I had gone through so many humiliating experiences, that I had held on to very little of my once overwhelming pride and self-esteem. After this experience, I had none left. In fact, if pride and dignity were held in my hand along with an old, tarnished penny, then it all added up to one cent. The good thing about this result is that these days, I do not get embarrassed—no matter what happens. But when my behavior oftentimes reflects an attitude of I really don't give a fat one whether or not you like me, because I gave it all at the hospital, my wife can get a little concerned that I might be offensive to others. And so if this writing offends you, then please refer back to the remains in my bedpan, now on display in the hospital hall of fame, and take a big bite!

After about two hours had passed after the toxic spill and clean up, I was shocked by a reoccurrence of the same event. Only this time, the nurse did not depend on Superman and when I told her she had eight seconds, she actually made it in seven. Needless to say, after about another half-hour of changing oil and lubing up the metal bedpan, The HAZMAT team reappeared and went through the entire process all over again. I don't know about you, but when several nurses pick up your legs and wipe you down like a baby with a poopy diaper except for the fact that you are a fully alert, and complete mind functioning middle-aged adult, and you are not wearing a diaper, but some metal device (bedpan) that originated somewhere back in the dark ages and was kept on through the era of enlightenment on to the wireless age of today, it is quite humiliating and it effects how you look at the world and your place in it. And ultimately, my rose-colored glasses kind of fogged over with a greenish hue.

After about three more sessions about an hour apart, the oil well stopped spouting for a time. In fact, a strange transition began to take place. The oil spout purged itself of lubricant and began to build up reserves of a translucent yellow-green watery substance. The best comparison I can come up with is Saudi Arabia meets Yellowstone National Park's Old Faithful geyser. And just like Old Faithful, the bubbling, boiling and churning water had to sit dormant for a while in order to build up enough steam pressure to spout off. Well after the HAZMAT team had retired for the day, and before the next spewage of steamy fluids from the bowels of the earth took place (figuratively speaking), I was able to make it through the night and survive to awaken on day six.

I began day six looking and feeling and smelling like a corpse that had just been dredged up out of a stagnate lake after a month of decomposition, bloating, and being nibbled at by the little lake creatures whose existence depended on their freshly found and very scarce food source. The basketball-sized tumor that now resembled the mutant growth sticking out of Arnold Schwarzenegger's mutant friend's chest in Total Recall hurt like hell, only you couldn't blast it into oblivion with a shotgun like in the movie, and any movement I made, no matter how careful, caused the turtle with the life support tube to shudder in pain. To make matters worse, I still couldn't eat and all I could drink was a little bit of the sweet apple nectar my wife was sneaking in to the room in her big purse.

(By the way, she is still a pro at smuggling things in her purse—especially drinks, sub sandwiches, burritos, pizza, candy, popcorn, a frozen yogurt machine, and a wide variety of other treats when we go to the movies. Come on, you all have done it a time or two so don't start pointing a finger at me. After all, how am I supposed to smuggle a water bottle or sub sandwich into the movies without bringing alarm sounding attention to my pant pockets?)

What I failed to realize in my dazed and weakened state, is that apple juice is a natural laxative, and Old Faithful was gathering steam. Now as far as my IV's were concerned, my hands and wrist had been poked and pierced so many times, that my hands began to swell up and be very painful. And, the IV's were not working well. And besides that, I had now lost so much blood that over the next three days, I would be receiving a blood transfusion each day of two pints of blood each time, and so it was critical that the IV's flowed well. Fortunately, after the first transfusion on day six, my vital signs started to stabilize enough to where the nurses gave me permission to get out of bed only when absolutely necessary. Or in other words, they were tired of wiping my butt and so I could go and do my business myself, even of the electrode signals from my chest spiked a little now and then. After all, there was a crash cart nearby and all of the staff had been well trained on how to use it. At this point, I felt so slimy, what I really wanted to do was go into a vacant room with concrete walls and floor, and just have someone hose me down with a fi re hose.

The procedure to get to the bathroom, which was only about six feet from my bed, had several steps involved. First, I had to carefully grab my catheter bag. Then, I had to get my two IV carts, one on each side of the bed, and carry all three items to the bathroom. There probably should have been a step in there to check and make sure that my body parts were modestly covered since the door to the hallway was open and looked directly toward my pathway to the john, but in all honesty, at this point of my stay, I could give a rat's behind who saw what. My face, greasy hair, and six day shadow, along with the blue bags under my eyes and the huge purple basketball would be so shocking that people would stare at my privates just for some visual relief. Once I arrived at the bathroom door, I would carefully hang the catheter bag on the inside door knob, make sure that I had enough slack in both IV tubes and that they were not tangled up so that any tension would not rip the IV's out of my plump, discolored, hole-ridden hands. Then, I could carefully go to the sink to wash up a bit or brush my teeth that now looked like one of Jack Sparrow's crew in Pirates of the Caribbean. I remember that on my first venture out of bed, I just shuffled into the bathroom, got a washcloth, ran it under very hot water, and just placed it on my face. The warmth felt as good as a hot shower after being rescued by the Coast Guard's Kevin Costner or Ashton Kutcher in the icy waters of northern Alaska in the movie "The Guardian."

After several washings, I returned back to the bed where my wife had just placed a newly purchased eggshell foam pad between my sheet and the mattress. Talk about deluxe accommodations! The nurse tried to tell her that it wasn't sanitary to have the pad under the sheets, but how can you take back a new puppy from your four-year old child on Christmas day because it sheds a little bit of hair on the carpet? That must have been the look on my face and my expression, along with my wife explaining that since my 30-gallon container of hazardous waste had by now been filled and disposed of at least five times, a little foam from Wal-Mart couldn't be that harmful. I just hoped that all of the unsupervised kids running around the store on past weekends had not opened my pad's package in the store and used it for a trampoline, facial wipe, and toilet.

Like I said before, getting out of bed was a real chore that took some time. Speaking of turtles, I felt like one it's back trying to move my arms and legs in pitifully slow gyrations until I could grab something to sit up. Then, I had to gently swing my legs over to the side while trying not to move the catheter tube. Next, I had to get the urine bag, clear the tube from catching on anything, and grab the IV cart attached to my left hand on the side of the bed opposite the bathroom and wheel it around to the bathroom side. Then, I had to grab the other IV cart attached to my right arm, make sure that the IV tubes did not cross. And finally, I had to rock back and forth until I had enough momentum to stand up. And if I were going to the bathroom, I had to carry and wheel everything over to the bathroom entrance, place my CB (catheter bag which I will refer to as this acronym from now on to save a lot of ink) gently on the inside of the door knob, park the IV carts at the entrance making sure that they did not become unplugged while still giving my hands enough tube so that the IV's didn't come out of my hands which now were all black and blue and looked like a pair of grape flavored rubber gloves that had been blown up to look like balloons with 5 stubs on the end. And after all this, I could then move on to take care of business. I would not describe this procedure in such detail if it weren't critical to the next part of the saga.

While in bed sometime during the midmorning of this, the sixth day, Old Faithful came out of dormancy with a vengeance like Hiroshima, except this time, no warning pamphlets dropped down from the ceiling to alert me to the impending explosion. And you must remember that my sphincter had gone AWOL to the extent that when he returned, he was sure to be court-martialed and shot at dawn for high treason. When the rectal panic attack occurred, the bedpan must have committed conspiracy with Mr. Sphincter, because he was nowhere to be found, yet I was confident that this time around, I could make it to the bathroom. I mean heck, it was only six feet away. It might just as well been located at an abandoned waste station off the coast of Iceland, for as soon as I stood up and there was any gravity force at all from my butt to my upper thigh, the trickling effect commenced so that by the time I had gone through the entire procedure and arrived at the bathroom door, my business was done. But, to save face, I sat down anyway—even if just to rest and to collect my thoughts as to what I was going to do next. As I looked down at the antifreeze on my legs and on the floor—which by the way left a fluorescent green stain for at least a month after I had gone home—I no longer had any concern over the sanitary status of my foam pad on the bed. To make matters worse, the damn toilet dispenser in the bathroom was like one of those you get in a cheap, open stall at a freeway rest stop that doesn't spin so you have to tear off one square at a time, or reverse roll the paper to be able to get several squares even though it inevitably rips anyway because the paper is so cheap.

Since I had nowhere to go at the time and all the time in the world to do nothing, I began to tear off squares of the cheap TP and make a neat pile on my thigh. After all, I needed to clean up the mess as best I could, and I just didn't have the guts to call out for the cleanup crew so soon after the recent episode. So I made my pile, got all my accessories together, and began to wipe up the radioactive trail of evidence I had left behind on my way to the porcelain throne. I did the best I could and slowly made it back into bed. I felt like a kid who had gotten into a five-pound bag of fl our and spread it all over the kitchen floor, walls, and furniture while mom was out of the room. I knew that I didn't have the capacity to clean it all up, but the little I did do partially absolved my guilty conscience.

What happened next was completely contrary to all reason since my diet was limited to the occasional sip of apple juice and a main course of ice chips. I was however indulging in bingeing myself with a smorgasbord of intravenous fluids containing a myriad of medicines, antibiotics, body fluids, vitamins, with a side order of blood transfusions that if all laid out, would fill more tables than the Circus, Circus buffet. As if I was in a reoccurring nightmare, I found myself in the middle of the Twilight Zone-like series of synchronized reruns and I mean literally reruns. I felt like I was the star in a very low-budget sequel of the movie Groundhog Day, and I was playing the character of Bill Murray. For the next three days, every half hour on the dot for an entire 24-hour period, and you could set your watch by my precision timing, I would experience this exact same procedure described above—right down to the very minute detail—which would repeat itself over and over and over again. The only thing I could be grateful for was that I did not have to listen to Sonny and Cher's "I Got You Babe" as the same episode continued to repeat itself. It was during this time that I realized that if I did not get out of there soon, this newly approved property of the Hotel California lodging franchise would be my final destination in life and I was sure that the conduit from this hellish realm to the next contained no bright light and tunnel ascending heavenward. I was convinced that if I passed on in this place, the only exit out went downward and was very hot, and I was to be escorted by demons like in the movie "Ghost," when the real bad guys realized that they were dead.

As the sun rose reflecting off of the shimmering stains down my leg on day nine, I was starting to get desperate. Unfortunately, I was on a very short and very secure leash—if you could call it that, in some sort of sick, demented sort of way. My abdomen was still bleeding and so my doctor ordered a CT scan to see if she could find out where the blood was coming from. Before I could do the CT scan the nurse cam in and asked me to drink a Super Big Gulp sized concoction of what tasted like lemon flavored Alka-Seltzer. I told her that there was no way I could drink it all and that the results could create a disastrous tidal wave of apocalyptic magnitude. She just smiled and told me that she knew I could do it and that everything would come out okay. I informed her of my problem and she assured me that any time we take in fluids, it takes about an hour for us to process them through our digestive tract before they can make it to the exit. I guess that she didn't realize what everything coming out okay actually meant, and I am certain that she had never before worked crowd control for a teen idol concert attended by crazed, adolescent, hormonally unbalanced teen-agers that explode when the rock star exits the limo toward the backstage entrance, but I reluctantly followed her orders anyway and drank the nasty stuff. When I was finished, I heard this rumbling noise equaling that of a rolling earthquake of epoch proportions on the rectum scale as I realized that the sound was coming from deep within my bowels. I knew that typically with an earthquake of that magnitude, A tsunami was sure to follow, and it was just a matter of time before the deluge struck.

Soon after I finished my beverage, the good old wheel chair guy (there were actually several that I was acquainted with by this point in my stay) got me in a wheel chair and took me, and all my gear to the elevator down to the Imaging Room. As we exited the elevator and were wheeling down the hallway, I could feel the tide going way out as the huge accelerating wave built up a churning undercurrent of sheer power in it's path of pending and certain destruction. I felt the cresting wall of fluids approaching and informed the wheel chair guy that we had to find a bathroom really quick. He reassured me that we could find one just as soon as we were finished with the scan. I think that he was just about to go on break and he didn't want to be delayed by any detour. Once again, my voice got quite agitated as I informed him that if we did not find a bathroom immediately, we would have a mess similar to the wall of blood rushing through the hallways in "The Shining." The wheel chair guy realized that it was either a quick detour or he was about to become a victim of a drive-by pooping. Fortunately, the hallway had a staff restroom. He rushed the door and pounded on it frantically. A female hospital staff member politely called out, "It's occupied, I'll be out in just a minute." My wheel chair guy having a sixth sense and realizing that the ticking time bomb only had a precious few seconds remaining before detonation, pounded on the door again and informed the female inside, "This is a medical emergency and we need to get in RIGHT NOW!" A few seconds later, a disgruntled nurse exited the bathroom while straightening her little frock decorated with some cute little cartoon animals on a sky blue background, and with a very bent out of shape expression on her face. Miraculously, I was able to make it all the way to the pot before I completely drained the fluids that were supposed to be present for the scan. After taking care of my business so completely and with maximum efficiency, I exited the potty and we continued down to do the scan. Fortunately, it was finished, and I was back to my room within a half an hour.

My surgeon came in to see me that afternoon and informed me that the CT scan did not reveal any vascular leakage. And after several consultations with other doctors, she decided that she was not going to open me back up to see if she could find the source of the bleeding. But, I would have to get my third two-pint blood transfusion. My vital signs had improved some, but they were still not within a safe range, and so I continued with the regimen of medications and fluids. The problem now was that both my hands and wrists were so swollen they could no longer use regular IV's. So, they scheduled me to go to X-ray to get a pick line placed in my upper arm so that they could give me the blood and other fluids now being restricted by swollen, bruised skin and veins that had retired to somewhere in South Florida for some R and R. The pick line is done by X-ray with the assistance of an X-ray machine so that the new line can be inserted into the main vein in the upper arm. Once successfully in place, the line was so big you could pump gasoline through that puppy! The procedure was a success and I was wheeled back to my room where all of the IV and blood bags were routed through one main line and hooked up to one IV cart. I am not sure how that cart didn't just topple over. It looked like a huge branch of ripened bananas. Anyway, it was working and as the night drew on, the blood and fluids flowed once again without restriction.

As the graveyard shift came on duty—and I use that term only now that the ordeal is over and most of the terror and post-traumatic shock syndrome symptoms have subsided, my new nurse introduced himself. His name was Ray and he was a very polite, soft-spoken guy from Philippine descent about 5 feet four inches tall weighing in at about I'd say 140 pounds or so. I describe him so that you know that at 6'5", weighing 275 pounds, I would be quite a handful for Ray to pick up if I were to fall. As he introduced himself, I asked him if he were good luck. With a slightly puzzled, yet pleasant look on his face he asked me why I asked. I told him straight out that he had to be good luck because I had to go home the next day for if I didn't, I knew that I was going to die there. He politely grinned as if to acknowledge my joke that wasn't really a joke at all but a desperate cry for help. He responded that he felt he was fairly good luck. I told him I needed a much more convincing reassurance that I would be able to go home that day, which had barely turned into day nine. I knew I had a long way to go before day nine was through, but I just had to have a light at the end of the tunnel in order to go on. He nodded his head and said, "Okay" whatever that meant and I took it as his way of confirming him as a real-life good luck charm. After all, I would take any sign at all as a positive one at this point.

I have not mentioned yet that my room was at the end of the hallway, I did not have any roommate, and the nurse's station was down at the beginning of the hallway. And besides my TV and my call button, at two o'clock in the morning the place was almost completely deserted and deathly quiet—the quiet before the storm. At two on the dot, I had my half-hourly urge to go. So, I hurriedly grabbed my bag and the banana branch loaded with IV's and took off to the bathroom with my usual sense of urgency. I just didn't have the strength to have my gown and bed sheets changed again. As I entered the bathroom, I quickly placed the urine bag on the doorknob and parked the IV cart outside the door. In my rush to get to the bottom of things, I vaguely remember noticing that the blood IV bags were now running on empty. By now, I was in a real hurry as the trickle-down effect was in motion.

At this point, I have to interject a bit of critical information in order to accurately explain what happened next. The hospital where I was staying is quite old. The staff was excellent as was my care, although they could have cleaned and sanitized the floor more often—especially the trail I had now blazed from my bed to the bathroom. In route, I knocked over the 30-gallon receptacle of hazardous waste material, sending debris of bandages, empty IV bags, and a whole lot of soiled jumbo wipes all over the room. Remaining focused on the ultimate goal, this small glitch was hardly a distraction at all. I visualized myself a running back in the NFL leaping over would be tacklers and somersaulting into the end zone. In reality, I was actually shuffling sideways, bent over with pain from my side and there was no way I could leap over a dime, let alone Brian Urlacher.

The fixtures in the bathroom were quite old and the toilet had an interesting accessory. Directly behind the middle of the toilet, there was a pipe with a nozzle on the end of it for cleaning purposes. This pipe was about 12 inches long and it was hinged so that the person doing the cleaning could bring it down to rinse the toilet or floor or whatever. However, over time this hinge had loosened up so that sometimes the pipe would slide forward, protruding out from the back of the toilet at about a 45 angle, where it would stay until someone pushed it back into place in a vertical position. Well as I rushed in to do my business, my checklist to that point had never included checking to make sure that the pipe was in it's upward and locked position. And so, as I frantically took a seat, I was impaled by the nozzle! And, instinctively reacting to the impalement and while falling backward, I threw my hands up into the air to catch my fall. When I did so, the pick line flew out of my arm and I found myself with blood spurting all over the walls, shit all over the floor, and a pipe sticking up my ass! (Sorry for the cuss words here but the story just doesn't have the same impact if I edit the words.)

My mind instinctively reverted back to my Boy Scout days when I studied first aid, which has been reinforced over the years by my CPR training for coaching at the high school level. As I took a quick glance around, I made a quick assessment of the situation to prioritize the next steps I needed to make. First, I realized that blood pumping out of my arm and into the air is not good—especially since I had just finished my third two-pint blood transfusion, so I knew I had to stop the bleeding or I would be facing another transfusion and three more comped nights at Hotel California. I immediately placed my hand over the wound—not my inflamed, hemorrhoid suffering anus which by now appeared quite similar to the dangling membrane protruding from the mother alien as she laid her army of eggs, but the hole where the pick line once was, and I applied direct pressure with my other hand. Once the bleeding was slowed with the pressure, I took a step forward to dislodge the pipe. Then I pushed the now tarnished pipe back into its upright and stowed position and sat down on the pot. My heart stopped racing and as I was able to focus my conscious awareness of what had just happened, I realized that my quick action had stopped the blood quite quickly, so I sat back maintain the direct pressure and thought about what to do next. As I looked over the devastation before me, I was amazed at how much damage a guy in my condition with all of the handicaps I had been shackled to, could do in such a brief period of time without any assistance whatsoever. If Hollywood were to recreate this scene, it would take stuntmen, explosives, miniature building and structural specialists, and about five different cameras giving different visual perspectives, and a host of support staff about a week to recreate. And yet I was able to do it all in one take and utilizing only the materials available in the room at the time.

All in all, I felt pretty darn accomplished! I had stopped the bleeding, contained the toxic refuse, removed the impaling post and I was now in a sitting position waiting for help. A key bit of information that I should interject here is that there is no telephone or call button in the bathroom. Apparently, no previous patient had experienced anything similar to what had just happened to me—go figure! And remember the location of my room and the hour of the day that this occurred. I figured that someone at some point would walk by, see the huge pile of spillage from the hazardous waste container, and peek in to see if I was still alive — heck, to investigate what appeared to be a visit from Jack the Ripper! I waited about ten minutes, placed some tissue squares on the wound, bent my arm to maintain the applied pressure, and then I guess out of force of habit, I started to make my little pile of TP squares. After I had a substantial pile and I had cleaned up some of the fluids of an assortment of colors and consistency, I decided to call out for help. I didn't want to sound panicky or desperate—especially so early in the morning when it was so tranquil, so I politely exclaimed, "Help!" "Is anybody out there?" "Help?" There was no response. I repeated the words with a bit more enthusiasm. Still no answer. I yelled a bit louder. Nothing.

After about 20 minutes or so, a large African American nurse walked by and glanced into my room. I only mention her race to provide you with a better visual representation of what actually occurred. Since I was sitting in the bathroom, I could not see her, but as soon as she looked in and saw what had to be a very disturbing scene, she ran inside the room and with enthusiasm and in a very piercing pitch, she exclaimed, "Oh my God!" "What happened here?" As she finished her verbal reaction, she turned her head into the bathroom where she saw me sitting on the pot, applying direct pressure on the wound, with a stack of neatly placed TP squares on my thigh and a somewhat contented look on my face. As our eyes met—hers much larger than mine—I said, "I had a little accident." She responded, "I can see that!" There was a brief awkward pause as we both thought of something to say to add to the interesting conversation. She went next. "Are you okay?" she asked. I nodded and said yes. Another pause. Then I spoke up next and asked her if she could get my nurse. She suddenly realized that this was her opportunity to escape and without hesitation she said, "I'll go get him right away!" and she took off sprinting down the hallway. I don't think I have ever seen a large woman run that fast before or since.

Soon after, Ray came in and looked over the situation and asked me what had happened. I said, "Well, I had a small accident and my pick line came out." He comfortingly responded with "I can see that," followed by, "let's get you cleaned up and back into bed." He brought me some jumbo wipes, a new gown, and helped me get back into bed. He assessed the situation and figured that although it looked pretty bad, I had not lost that much blood, so I didn't need a new pick line, as long as he could find a vein in my hand to attach the IV tubes. He strapped two rubber tourniquets to my arm and somehow coaxed a vein out of hiding amidst the carnage long enough to get a line through and he started up the IV's again. I have always believed that something good comes out of adversity, and this time there was no exception. My theory is that the shock of the event to my system caused my blood to coagulate in some way as to stop my internal bleeding because from the moment of impalement, the drainage stopped. Or, perhaps the pipe lodged in so deep that it put pressure on the leaking vessel and caused it to stop. All I know is that from that moment, I began to stabilize, and the internal healing intensified.

I informed Ray at that very moment that I was going to go home that day no matter what, or I would die trying—which was probably more likely to happen. He just smiled, nodded and said, "Well, we'll see." I reminded him that he was good luck and that it would happen. He smiled again, said good night, and turned out the light for me to get some sleep. I will say that my wife was in my room all day, each day, unless she had errands to run. And I hold no ill feelings toward her for not sleeping in a chair in my room that night. And I am glad that she didn't, as the whole scene may have been too much for her to take.

The next morning, I announced to the new nurse coming on duty that I wanted to see my surgeon and that I would be going home that day—day 9 still. Nurses sure have the line "We'll see" down pat, as this was her response as well. I wondered if Ray had conspired against me at the change of shift meeting. To prepare myself for the big interview, I actually asked for a shower room to primp up. I was given a small room with a shower, sink and toilet, along with a complimentary deluxe hygiene kit, including generic toothpaste and a toothbrush, which was literally that, one very coarse stout hair on a plastic brush. In fact, I bet this hair came from someone's ear that resided in the nearby geriatrics ward. I took a very long, hot shower. I also shaved with the deluxe single-blade razor and sample sized shaving crème that would never even make it to the clearance rack at the local 99-cent store. With the very cheap razor, I shaved off my week and a half shadow along with a layer of skin, and applied the medicated hand lotion from the dispenser on the sink for the only after-shave available, and as a blood coagulant. I felt better but still looked like hell. As I looked at my emaciated face in the mirror, the realization that I had lost some weight was obvious. (In fact, upon my final return home, I weighed myself to find that I had lost 25 pounds in nine days. It is the most successful diet I have ever been on. I have even thought about getting the "Gall Bladder Diet" published in the Enquirer or other reputable magazine.) I cinched up my gown, closed the butt flap on the back—which opened right back up as soon as I took a step, and wheeled my IV cart back to my room to await my visitors.

My surgeon finally came in around lunchtime and I shared my previous night's experience with her. She had a good laugh at my expense. I joined in on the laughter. We had to have a connection going when I popped the question. So, I asked her if I could go home today and told her that bad things were happening and that if I didn't leave that very day, I was convinced I would die that very day. She told me that she would like to see me eat some solid food first. I asked her if she had ever eaten at that hospital before and she responded that doctors get their food at this hospital for free. I said, "You didn't answer the question. Have you actually eaten the food here?" She grinned, nodded her head and said that she had. I told her that someone from food services had finally offered me some solid food that day, and they brought in baked fi sh at about ten thirty in the morning. Now I don't know about you but I was not about to eat hospital fish when their Jell-O tasted like what was mopped up from my bathroom earlier that day. I told her that what I needed was to get the tube out of the turtle, go home to finally get some rest, and eat some of my wife's food, not the food of some guy who received his culinary training at Singh-Singh. She chuckled and said she'd see what she could do. She also told me that the hospital's attending doctor who originally admitted me also had to approve my release. I told her to do what she had to do in order to make it happen.

Remember I told you that I put my faith in divinity while at the hospital. Well, my faith was about to once again be put to the ultimate test. My surgeon had signed my release. Then it was time for my second interview with the attending physician. She entered my room early in the afternoon of day nine. As she entered, I felt a blast of hot, sweaty air as if she had traveled through a portal from the underworld of Hades itself. The portal quickly closed in behind her, holding back a host of demons pushing desperately toward the momentary escape hatch. She acknowledged that there was a good possibility for me to go home that day. I let out a silent scream! Then came a blow that would have felt like a blow to the testicles—except they had long since gone into deep hiding. She told me that she was still very concerned that I would be able to urinate on my own and that she would release me to go home that day if the catheter came along with me. The news brought on a shock wave so deep within me that it dislodged the testicles so that they free fell until they finally struck rock bottom at about knee height! I pleaded with her that taking it with me defeated the purpose of granting me freedom as I would still be chained to this heavy load that made Jacob Marley's chains look like an ankle bracelet. I further explained that I hadn't slept now for over three days and that I really needed to sleep and it was impossible to do so with barbed wire up my now emaciated private part. Somewhere through the process of my passionate pleas, her heart softened. Her change of heart was as miraculous as the transformation of the Grinch, and as astonishing as the last act of compassion by Darth Vader to save the life of his son Luke from his pending demise at the hands of the evil emperor.

She made a deal with me. She said that if I could prove that I could pee on my own, then she would have the razor blade riddled hose removed. Further, I had to swear that if I was plugged up at home and if my stomach became bloated from the buildup of impassable urine, that I would promise to immediately go to the emergency room and have them reinsert the beast for a fourth time. I had no choice but to agree to her term's conditional surrender. So, the nurse came in to remove the catheter for hopefully the final time—and I mean final as I seriously would have died of a toxic urine overdose rather than go back to the hospital for another round of POW torture. And so, just as if the windows of heaven opened wide and a myriad of guardian angels swooped down to save my anguished soul, the nurse came in to remove the device. My breathing to distract from the discomfort was replaced by my cries of pure ecstasy as she deflated the bulb and removed the tube. The turtle opened his eyes ever so slightly as the removal acted like life regenerating electric shocks purging through my body like the paddles from a crash cart defibrillator.

I saw the light at the end of the tunnel—either that or a tunnel of light leading to heaven. Either way, a feeling of euphoric liberation came over me. From deep within my very being came a Richter-registering shudder of delight and relief. Just imagine that you have stood in line to see the premiere showing of a movie's release and that you have awaited this event for over six months. Then as you watch the movie with your popcorn and large drink, even though you will never finish it but you bought it because it was the best value, and right at the climax of the movie, you have to go to the bathroom. But since you can't miss a single moment and you contemplate peeing in the big movie beverage cup but your conscience convinces you not to go through with it as you are surrounded by strangers and they may hear the splashing in the cup during a brief moment of silence, you wait until the end of the movie and sprint to the bathroom where you set a new record for the Guinness Book of World Records for the longest continuous flow and the most volume of urine ever, and you shudder with pure delight and relief. Well, multiply that feeling times a thousand and you can imagine the feeling that I experienced.

Then immediately following the removal, she handed me the plastic pee bottle and told me to go and gather some evidence. I have to admit that I was a bit nervous that I could perform, especially since the nurse had just emptied the bag that was full to the brim. As I started to get out of bed, I spotted the apple juice that my wife had brought me and I figured that if things got desperate, I could resort to devious means of falsifying the sample. But, I thought that I would try to do it the natural way to avoid getting caught by the hidden cameras that I was certain were placed in any private area where I could relieve myself with the live monitors manned by vigilant security guards who had been instructed to watch me and make sure that I made my own pee. So, I went into the now historic bathroom, which had been cleaned out by a custodial staff who was at that very moment in the hospital administration office demanding a raise and raised the bottle into position. Remember when I mentioned my ultimate test of faith in divine powers? Well standing there in the solitude of the hospital can, I uttered the sincerest and heart-wrenching prayer of my life pleading with heavenly intervention to open up my freshly rerouted plumbing.

As I exerted what little pressure I could as the pain in my bruised abdomen throbbed with any kind of pressure, and with my rectum instinctively reacting to the push, my memory of this procedure that had been automatic for so many years was refreshed into my mind as I took the steps to complete the process. No less miraculous than a faith healing of a wheelchair imprisoned, acutely arthritic invalid as they rise up from their chair and walk until they collapse into a spiritual stupor onto the stage, the urine trickled out. I too, let out a hallelujah and approached the very edge of passing out, as I lifted the goblet of life as the baboon witch doctor lifted up the newly born future lion king. There wasn't a lot of liquid, but there was enough. I thought about supplementing it with some juice, but my Freudian Super Ego convinced the Ego to not give in to the devilish urges of my Id, and I didn't give in to the urge.

(Freud had some pretty strange ideas but hey, I teach Psychology remember?) Like the Special Forces soldier who carefully poured the nitroglycerin into the explosive device that would free the hostages being held by gunpoint by terrorists, I carefully delivered the evidence to my nurse, and proudly lifted the prized fluids. And to my astonishment and sheer joy, I was absolved from my gall bladder's sins and released from captivity.

I said my good-byes promising I would never return alive—which in the years ahead became an outright lie many times over. My wife pulled the van around to the exit and I was wheeled for the last time by the wheel chair guy out to the van. He locked the brakes, came around the front and removed my feet from the little foot pedals. Fortunately, my feet were sporting the latest in designer hospital footwear. They were covered with those little socks with the anti-slip strips that were about three sizes too small—but hey, who cares? Heck, I would have streaked down the hall and out into the parking lot and on through the middle school adjacent to the hospital if it would have meant my release. Fortunately, all I had to do was get out of the chair and into the van for the short ride home.

"Free at last, free at last." "Thank God Almighty—free at last!" Now as I repeat this famous quote by Martin Luther King, you must understand that I mean absolutely no disrespect whatsoever. Its just that as I was released from the medical chains of bondage and wheeled through the outer doors of this "correctional institution," I felt the liberating freedom only experienced by those who have shared in this moment of coming out of the darkness of strict confinement and into the light of sovereignty, and these words came to my mind as I exclaimed my praises of rejoicing heavenward!

After I got home, it took a month for me to be able to eat solid food. And I had lost any appetite for sweets, chocolate, and colas (even though unfortunately the cravings for sweets and chocolate has returned with a passion). I couldn't eat any spicy or rich or fatty foods. In other words, by sheer necessity, my body had reverted to eating a healthy diet, which I had not done since I was weaned off of Gerber's. As a result, I learned a great lesson trough this whole crisis. The lesson is quite simple. Our body is an amazing machine. When something goes wrong, our body sends out warning messages. All we have to do is listen to the warnings and take action to ensure that the problems are corrected. If we do so, we will live a much happier and much longer life.

After about three weeks, I was able to return to work—although I was all clammy and looked like death warmed over. The bruise dissipated and disappeared after about two months. Over the next three months, I ended up losing about 40 pounds. Another post-surgery symptom I had acquired brought my very gender into question for the very first time, as I began to pass through menopause. From the moment I arrived home, I began to experience hot flashes—especially during the night when I would get so hot, that I would have to get out of bed and lay down in front of a big fan in the family room. And, even then, my head would get so hot that I had to place an icepack under my pillow and keep turning it over to the cool side to try and get some sleep. For about four months, I averaged about four hours of sleep a night. Because, like a radiator with a blown thermostat, my head would boil over with heat and sweat. And to this day, I still have a problem sleeping through the night and I cannot sleep in like I used to.

One noteworthy side note here is that after I was home for several weeks, I went to see my surgeon for my post-operation follow-up visit. As I mentioned earlier, I brought her flowers and she took our picture. All went well at the check up until the very end when she hit me with a groin shot I can best compare to an experience I had while coaching high school freshman softball several years ago.

During practice one day, I decided to pitch for batting practice. Usually, we have a pitching machine do the pitching and all I had to do is feed the machine with softballs and it would do the rest. And to be safe with the machine, I stood behind a safety net to protect myself from the batters as they swung away. Well this time, we were on a practice field without any power to plug in the machine, so I decided it would be okay to go ahead and pitch myself. And, since I can't pitch real fast, I assumed that the velocity of the ball coming off the bat would also be slower, so I figured that a safety net would not be necessary. Everything was going fi ne until our clean-up batter, a girl who led our team on home runs over the fence, approached the little make shift rubber home plate. I was pitching underhanded and so my pitches were not very fast, and I kept them slow to keep up what little control I had at getting the pitches over the plate. After she had hit several screamers, I wound up and gave her a big fat strike right over the plate. And, just like a precisioned submarine torpedoist, she launched a warhead with the trajectory of a lethal direct hit at the heart of the enemy vessel. As the projectile found it's mark, I found new meaning for the term, "scrambled eggs," as some of my testicular vessels ruptured and I dropped like a rock! Now mind you when this happened, I was surrounded by 15 high school softball girls. However, upon impact, the last thing on my mind was to protect my male ego by attempting to ignore what had just happened. At this point, I had no control whatsoever over my evolutionary instinct to drop and cover, which I did even though the cover part was way too late. As I lay there observing the fourth of Julyesque fireworks show, I held back my internal defense mechanism manifested by a strong wave of nausea and overwhelming desire to vomit, and only allowed a gag refl ex to show itself to preserve what little manhood I had left. As I slowly came to my senses and tenderly rose to my feet (still doubled over), I must have done so quite pathetically as several girls offered to help me get up. In fact, the blow was so intense, that even these very typical high school girls did not laugh—at least until I acknowledged that I was okay. As I took a big breath and exhaled a frail, raspy "I'm okay," we all let out a brief chorus of nervous laughter that sounded more like sympathy than humor. I very quickly realized that there was no way that I could finish the hitting drill, let alone the rest of practice, so I asked the freshman coach if he could hold and supervise a little scrimmage between the two teams as I had to leave due to unexpected circumstances that needed my immediate and complete attention. So, I gingerly bent over and picked up my glove, my pride, and what was left of my eggs (English for juevos, the Spanish word for eggs that also refers to testicles—isn't Spanish so much more of an expressive language than English?) which once fi t snugly in the enclosed eggshell but were now shattered and scrambled, whipped and pureed, and limped to my car and drove home, where I laid down for the rest of the evening with an icepack on my privates and a Band-Aid on my manhood.

To make a long story a bit longer, the groin shot by my surgeon was that I had to have another ERCP to remove the tube that was inserted on the first ERCP prior to removing the gall bladder. So, after about a month of nervous fretting, I decided to face my fears and I called Lucifer to schedule the removal of the tube. I was scheduled for the ERCP and this time, I was determined to inform all medical staff members involved in the follow up procedure that I was a big guy, that I had built up quite a resistance to pain medications, and that I absolutely did not want to be alert during the removal of the tube. I remember to this day telling every staff member on duty that day that I wanted to be completely knocked out this time around. I even told the custodians to inform the doctor that I wanted a very generous amount of the anesthetic so that I would not be awake like the last time. I reminded the nurse who put in my IV, the nurses that wheeled me into the surgery room, the assisting team, and yes, I even informed Satan as soon as he entered the room that I was the guy who was fully awake the last time. He must have remembered and I am comforted with the knowledge that even Satan at times—or at least once—showed some compassion and knocked me out before proceeding to remove the stint. All I remember from the incident is being wheeled into the operating room, while pleading for my life, and awaking in the recovery room with the procedure now behind me.

I will end the chapter by saying this. I am glad to be alive and that I survived to share his tale with whomever reads it. Let it serve as a beacon of warning, comfort, and humor to all humanity as we all pass through this experience we call life.

Chapter 6

A Colonoscopy Is Kind of Like a NASA Apollo Moon Launch...

My doctor, or should I say my physician's assistant that works for my primary care physician, had been telling me for years that when I turned 50, I would need to schedule a colonoscopy. This is a word that floats around out there but is seldom discussed in detail. I know what colon means and I know what scope means, so as I combine these two words into one, they basically mean that the doctor is going to insert a periscope up my rectal cavity. And, the closer I approached the golden age of 50, the more inquiries I made and the more I confirmed my definition. However, hearing the details are just not the same as going through the experience, just as watching the devastation of a train wreck on television is not the same as being on the train. And since I have given away the basic idea of the procedure, I thought that I would take a different approach to explaining the experience by comparing it to a NASA Apollo moon launch instead. In order to do this, I am going to illustrate the procedure with vocabulary typically associated with NASA. I will list the terms in a somewhat sequential order and follow them up with an explanation of the term relative to my own launch experience.

1.   Pre-Flight Checklist: For once and quite ironically, the approval process through my HMO took nothing more than a phone call to my doctor. Soon after, I received the referral and was requested to call the doctor's office to schedule the rectal photo session—more like involuntary colon violating rape kit including some KY Jelly and a very rough two by four. As I

read the name of the doctor on the referral, my sphincter quivered and I knee-jerk responded with a series of dry heaves. The doctor was the same one who performed the ERCP during my gall bladder episode at the hospital. You remember—Dr. Satan, Son of Darkness! I inquired if there were any other doctors on the approved list, but as fate would have it, his name was the only one. It was as if the medical group had slipped in a "Sign Your Soul Over to the Devil for Eternity In Return For Your Extended Life" form to sign along with the other piles of paperwork and disclaimers and full disclosure and privacy law papers that I had to fill out in order to receive any treatment whatsoever. With absolutely no alternative and after taking a considerable amount of time contemplating the possibility of having to pass through agonizing and potentially lethal colon cancer rather than seeing Lucifer again, I gave his office a call and scheduled the procedure. During the phone call, I was informed that I would be receiving a prescription in the mail and that I was to follow a very careful list of instructions that accompanied the RX, the failure of which would result in the postponement of the procedure to a future date.

2.   Rocket Fuel: As the fateful day approached, I received the prescription which was to be filled and ingested 24 hours prior to the colonoscopy, which I will refer to as the CS from here on out. I had heard from friends who had gone through with a CS before, that I would be taking some medication that would clean me out. What they didn't tell me was that as a result of the clean out, my colon would be so spotlessly shiny, that even Mr. Clean could see his reflection in it! At the time, all I know is that when the pharmacist passed me the container through the drive-up window, it barely fit in the sliding

compartment. As she passed it through to me after I had already signed and paid for it so that I couldn't request a substitute or refund for obsolete dark-age remedies right up there with blood-letting and crocodile dung, I had no choice but to accept the gallon-sized plastic container and take it home for further examination, explanation, and contemplation. Before I left, the pharmacist came to the window to explain directions so that I couldn't claim ignorance on the day of the CS. I was told that I was to fill the container all the way to the top, and shake it well so that the powder inside would dissolve completely in the water. Then, I was to drink 10 ounces every ten minutes until the entire two leaders were gone, which would last about 90 minutes. I did ask if the powder had a pleasant flavor to it. I was informed that it tasted kind of lemony. I guess that that explanation was provided by someone who saw the glass as half full. Otherwise, I would have been give the description of flavor to be compared to something like, oh I don't know, like a very liquidy turd from someone who had just downed a big glass of lemonade. So, I took the container home as I reflected on the upcoming event, and just as a top-ranked prizefighter would do prior to a title fight, I began the process of psyching myself up for the main event about to take place.

3.   All Systems Go For Launch: I returned home and commenced the countdown for launch. I changed into my space suit which was not of NASA issue, but just some loosely fitting gym shorts with a generous elastic waste and stretchable drawstring for quick removal. I filled the jug with water and I even added some Crystal Light lemonade for flavoring, recognizing that the pharmacist hesitated just for a moment and averted any eye contact when she deceitfully informed me

of the "lemony" flavor at the time of the purchase. Then, I measured out ten ounces of water into a glass as a practice round, so that I would know how much of the liquid nitro I would have to pour into the glass once the "All Systems Go For Take Off" had officially commenced. I sat down in my lounge chair with the jug, the glass, and my favorite show DVRed the night before and got as comfortable as possible. I checked the reclining mechanism in my chair to make sure that it could open and close without too much difficulty. This procedure reminded me of The Green Mile when the guards did a practice run on Old Sparky to make sure that the process of an actual execution would run smoothly. I checked my watch to synchronize the time with the instruction sheet that accompanied the jug, and I commenced the official countdown. As you are probably aware, once the countdown has begun, a critical stage is reached that I will call The Point of No Return when the mission can no longer be aborted. I had now reached that point in time of the launch sequence. It was as if the Commander in Chief and the Secretary of Defense had both simultaneously scanned their handprints and retinas, turned their keys, entered the proper sequence of numbers, and pushed the big red button to commence fi ring the nuclear warhead that would begin World War III and mark the beginning of the end—Armageddon. It was time. The end was literally near. I poured the glass. I bent over, kissed my still intact ass good-bye, and downed the first ten-ounce glass. I have never before felt such a sudden, instantaneous, and violent reaction as I did as soon as I ingested the liquid nitro. It had no sooner hit my stomach, when the turbulent caldron erupted into a violent inverted tornado spiraling downward with unimaginable velocity and destructive force that gives further meaning to the term, "blast off."

4. Strapping In, Launching Pad, and Lift Off. I will combine these three terms, as they are inseparable as far as what happened next. I have seen all the astronaut movies. I know that once ignition takes place and lift off commences, everything starts to shake and tremble and the propelling explosion causes complete incineration of the launching pad and surrounding areas. My case was no different except for one little procedural step that I could not have foreseen, and so failed to plan for. Looking back in retrospect, I know now that I should have somehow had seat belts installed into the side of the seat, or into the floor underneath. The problem with that is how can you go to Home Depot and ask them for a seat belt kit for your toilet? It's kind of like going to Victoria's Secret and asking if they have any slinky nightgowns for men. (Don't worry—I have never done this and when it comes to intimate apparel, I always tell my wife to surprise me and buy something nice that she would like. I just get nervous going into those stores. Like I said, I much prefer Home Depot and power tools, but saying it like that, you could still get the wrong idea about me.) I spend a lot of time at Home Depot as it is one of my favorite stores, and yet I have never seen anything resembling a retrofitting kit for this type of unconventional bathroom fixture. And, frankly, I would be quite embarrassed to ask the cute girl that works in the bathroom fixture section of the store for something quite so intimate as a toilet seatbelt. But now looking back on it, any humiliation resulting from the question would be far outweighed by the practicality and necessity of this type of addition. And, I firmly believe that as the average age of home depot workers surpasses the 50-year-

old mark, this idea will not only be implemented, but that they will even put up a header sign for the newly named isle called "Accessorizing for Your Colonoscopy!" At the time, if I had the courage to have overcome my embarrassment and done so, perhaps lift off would not have been so destructive. However, since I failed to take this precautionary measure, lift off was quite literally and without exaggeration just that—lift off. I had heard it said many times before the scientific law that for every action, there is an equal and opposite reaction, but I never really understood the law as it applies to real-life experience. In retrospect, I now have a greater insight into this law because as a result of the violent action, permanent evidence of the opposite and equal reaction was the embedded imprint of my footprints that remained in the concrete as an after effect of lift off. I had learned firsthand that the accessories isle in Home Depot would also include a concrete reinforcement kit to withstand the reactionary force of lift off. This kit would provide the added stability without which, the trajectory of the porcelain ship could shift to a horizontal trajectory which would have shot me out the door and down the hallway on my way to a crash landing with catastrophic results.

5. Sonic Boom: Ever since I was a little kid, I have heard sonic booms when Air Force jets fly overhead. And, I have seen the movie and read the book called, "The Right Stuff" about Chuck Yeager breaking the sound barrier but reading about it or hearing it from thousands of feet away is just not the same thing as being in the cockpit of the aircraft at the time of the boom! The sounds I heard and the ensuing shock wave that hit me shook me to my very core. I have never felt such a contrasting dichotomy of simultaneous sensations and emotions as I did at that moment of release. It was the best of

times, it was the worst of times. I felt intense horror, yet utter relief. I experienced unimaginable discomfort, yet immense release; reverberating shock, yet an unrestrained gush. The sound was deafening and the hyper-drive drainage quite unnerving. The shock wave accompanying the tidal wave of debris had a mushroom cloud effect similar to an atomic blast, sending a cloudy mass that exploded upward and outward reaching even the remotest of virgin porcelain yet to be exposed to any source of imaginable (or even unimaginable) expelled bodily fluids. The experience was almost a surreal, out of body episode where it appeared as if my spiritual entity had been temporarily exiled from my mortal shell to remain floating in the air while I waited for the opportune moment to reenter my body and expel the demon who had violated my soul. The occurrence was brief, yet profoundly intense.

I must say that those Europeans sure have one up on us in the personal hygiene department with their bidets as standard equipment in all homes and apartments. Unfortunately, this is not Europe and I had no bidet nor garden hose available, so I did the best I could to clean up the mess—at least the part that had blown up my back side. As I flushed, I tried not to look—and I know you can relate to the urge to check out your business, so don't act so shocked or offended! In fact, one time my son took a picture of his masterpiece with his cell phone and showed it off to his friends as if he had just won a trophy or something. So, as I flushed, I instinctively peeked at my work. That was a big mistake! The vivid memory has been permanently imprinted in my brain. I can best compare this to watching "The Exorcist" for the very first time with my friends at a sleepover when I was a kid. I had to at least pretend to be brave since covering my eyes in front of my peers would have exposed me as a wimp. So, I had no choice but to keep my eyes open while Linda Blair performed the 360-degree rotation of her head while barfi ng pea soup, levitating off of her bed and cussing out the priest with a voice sounding like Darth Vader with throat cancer. I will never forget the vivid memory of both of these traumatic events in my life. After the shocking peek that convulsively resulted in a double take that I regretfully cannot take back either, I gingerly walked back to my lounge chair in hopes that I could begin to watch the recording of my favorite TV show—or at least one segment in between commercials. Silly me! I barely had time to reach for the remote. As soon as I went to sit down, my upper torso bent over to an approximate 90-degree angle, as if in a squatting position, and spasmodically, my bowels followed suit in domino-style synchrony as the flood gates from the second 10-ounce glass spun uncontrollably wide open. Since my sphincter had finally returned from his AWOL status and with no replacement recruit available for the job, his status was reinstated to active duty and called to immediate service! Fortunately for me, his conditioned ability to instantly react and respond to an emergency situation of imminent danger from his previous extensive tour of duty, gave him the instinctive ability to delay the explosion until I could shuffle my way back down the green mile and plop down on Old Sparky. If Old Sparky could somehow magically talk, I'm sure that he would express an unexpected surprise to see someone so anxious to sit down on his lap and beg for an immediate lethal dose of electricity!

6.   G-Force: The dictionary defines G-force as "a unit of force equal to the force exerted by gravity; used to indicate the force to which a body is subjected when it is accelerated." A

dictionary of applied science explains horizontal g-force in this way: *Aircraft, in particular, exert g-force along the axis aligned with the spine. This causes significant variation in blood pressure along the length of the subject's body, which limits the maximum g-forces that can be tolerated. In aircraft, g-forces are often towards the feet, which forces blood away from the head; this causes problems with the eyes and brain in particular. As g-forces increase brownout/greyout can occur, where the vision loses hue. If g-force is increased, further tunnel vision will appear, and then at still higher g, loss of vision, while consciousness is maintained. This is termed "blacking out". Beyond this point loss of consciousness will occur, sometimes known as "G-LOC" ("loc" stands for "loss of consciousness"). While tolerance varies, a typical person can handle about 5 g (49m/s²) before g-loc. But through the combination of special g-suits and efforts to strain muscles—both of which act to force blood back into the brain— modern pilots can typically handle 9 g (88 m/s²) sustained (for a period of time) or more (see High-G training). Resistance to "negative" or upward g's, which drive blood to the head, is much lower. This limit is typically in the -2 to -3 g (-20 m/s² to -30 m/s²) range. The subject's vision turns red, referred to as a red out. This is probably because capillaries in the eyes swell or burst under the increased blood pressure.*

You may get a bit lost in this scientific description as I did, so let me just say this, and I will say it in very plain English for all to understand, using some key terms from the above explanation. As far as g-force is concerned in my colon-cleansing pre-procedure preparation, I know for a fact that I experienced blood draining from my head, tunnel vision, brown-out, grey-out, red-out, inside-out, and a definite swelling and bursting of the capillaries in my eyes so that they looked as big as those of Homer Simpson! Unfortunately, however, I did not experience G-LOC, as I was awake although quite disoriented during the entire purging.

7. Gravitational Pull: I know that Sir Isaac Newton was the guy who came up with the theory of gravity. However, I also know that gravity has always existed—it is a law of nature. I also have done a little research to know that the formula for gravitational pull is scientifically explained something like this:

$$F = G\frac{m_1 m_2}{r^2},$$

(Every point mass attracts every other point mass by a force pointing along the line intersecting both points. The force is proportional to the product of the two masses and inversely proportional to the square of the distance between the point masses where:
- F is the magnitude of the gravitational force between the two-point masses,
- G is the gravitational constant,
- m_1 is the mass of the first point mass,
- m_2 is the mass of the second point mass,
- r is the distance between the two-point masses.)

To me, this is a bunch of nonsense. I really have no clue as to the science of gravity and so I have come up with a formula of my own that would describe my experience with intestinal gravity based upon my drinking the two liters of diuretics. That formula looks something like this:

¥ [? /   X   *%#@!!!

Which is interpreted as: **A Pre-colonoscopy blow out is one violent SOB!!!**

8. Thrusters and Retro-Rockets: Thrusters are small rocket engines located around the orbiter's nose that maneuver the orbiter in space. I could say that the human thrusters I utilized during my circular orbit around planet "Your Anus" functioned in a similar fashion. The main difference to me is

that my thrusters operated completely on instinct. The thrusters of an Apollo spacecraft functioned as part of a well-synchronized, intricate plan of sequenced events to bring about a precise orbital positioning. On the other hand, or in this case as I figuratively turned the other cheek, my thrusters were completely spontaneous and quite convulsive in nature. Their major function was to fi re out rapid bursts of flaming fuel in order to stabilize my orbit around the toilet bowl by keeping my vertical positioning in a perpendicular plane from the surface of the toilet.

Retro-rockets are used in a lunar landing to slow the lander's speed of descent prior to hitting the surface. My retro, or should I say rectal rockets were on a very necessary manual override during my landing mission. The reason being quite simple: if anything at all had interfered with my rapid speed of descent prior to hitting the porcelain surface, the result would have been disastrous! The debris alone that would have been discharged from the lunar module would have caused such a scene of carnage and destruction, that if this landing site was previously known as the Sea of Tranquility, it would now have to be renamed Shipwrecked Island—with a little change in spelling by changing the letter "p" in Ship, to the letter "t."

9.   Splashdown: With the space program, splashdown occurs when a space capsule reenters the earth's atmosphere at a very specific mathematical rate of return, taking into consideration both gravity and drag to ensure the safe arrival of the craft and crew. My splashdown was a non-mathematical based occurrence that had complete disregard for both gravity and drag. Demons from hell were the only control room support staff. With no regard for life or limb, they engaged full power from every stomach and intestinal control system

available as they defiantly ensured no such safe arrival or controlled velocity of the payload. Their only desire was to create total chaos by initiating all launch systems for the entire bowel system's arsenal of rockets, missiles, or any other form of rectile projectile from scientific vessels to weapons of mass destruction at their disposal. The aftermath of such destruction would have been no less devastating had it been global nuclear war. After all, my world as I knew it, would never, ever be the same as a result of this abdominal Armageddon.

10. Asteroid Storm: Word derivatives formed by the root words ass and rhoids, thus creating the term ass-storm of hemorrhoidal proportions, or asteroid storm for short. Need I say more? I didn't think so.

11. De-Orbit Burn: The de-orbit burn in a spacecraft is completed by fi ring the orbiter's engine to slow its speed and take it out of orbit. Using the engines, the orbiter is turned around so that it is moving backwards at a slower speed, to allow a proper angle of re-entry and descent to direct most of the aerodynamic heating to the larger underside of the vehicle where the heat resistant tiles give the greatest amount of protection. The de-orbit burn that occurs during the purging of the diarrhetic solution is conceptually similar. My de-orbit burn operational definition is that when the orbiter (your anus) is desperately moving backwards and downwards making an extremely rapid decent at re-entry into the toilet bowl atmosphere to contain the discharge of fluids that could overflow and cause catastrophic collateral damage over the entire bathroom floor, walls, and fixtures, the anal cavity located on the underside of your backside re-enters the porcelain first, thus allowing the largest portion of the buttocks the greatest exposure to the intense heat and friction caused by

re-entry. Unfortunately, we have no heat resistant tiles that give us any amount of protection whatsoever, and so the underside of our anatomy is fully exposed to the extreme incineration that leaves a conduit of scar tissue and inflamed membrane manifested in a scarring vapor trail all the way down a hemorrhoid so engorged that you can funnel it down your pant leg and tuck it into your sock.

12. Hubble Telescope: The Hubble Telescope was carried into orbit by the space shuttle Discovery. It is the largest, most versatile telescope ever designed to be serviced in space by astronauts. It is well-known as both a vital research tool and a public relations boon for astronomy. In contrast, the colonoscopy camera is a small fi ber optic video camera on a flexible tube that is neither vital in rectal research nor a public relations boost for proctology.

In order to get a clear visual picture of the colon, the colon is first purged from any and all debris and then inflated with air to get a clear picture. It can provide a visual diagnosis that can be followed up with the biopsy or removal of any suspected lesions. I realize that this is an important preventative measure that can provide for early detection of colon cancer, and I do not want to offend anyone or make light of such an important procedure. But on the other hand, how can you keep a straight face while discussing a complete blow out of your bowels followed by filling your rectum up with air and taking pictures of the inside of your colon? If I were to come up with a theme song for the event, I can think of several candidates. For one, I can think of "Up, Up, and Away, In My Beautiful, My Beautiful Balloon." I also think of "Pop Goes the Weasel," and one more of many musical selections that come to mind is "Stop, In the Name of Love." But all in all I am grateful that the anesthesiologist gave in to my pleading for an extra dose of tranquilizers because I don't remember any of the exact details, but I do vaguely remember a few pokes and prods, and then I have a pretty good recollection of the colon deflation process which I used as an excuse for the following two to three weeks to justify farting around my wife in bed or walking down the hallway or even riding in the car as I reminded her that I was just following the doctor's orders to rid my system of unwanted gas. Ultimately, I had to give up on that excuse to fart and reverted back to complaining of the need to fart due to digestive problems as a result of her bad cooking. Both excuses ended up with the same result of giving me a "time out," or placing me on restrictions from any form of intimate activities. Oh well, at this age, a good dish of ice cream or some Oreo's and ice-cold milk are just as satisfying and the refractory period, better known as replacing the good old lead in the pencil., or replacing the lead in the good old pencil, however you want to put it, takes a lot less time. I have found that I can have unlimited feelings of passionate ecstasy with every bite of ice cream, or every dunked cookie without any delay whatsoever. And on top of that, I am a bit lactose intolerant so that the milk and the ice cream add to my chronic gas condition which compounds the problem so that over time, I eat much more cookies and milk and ice cream than I have intimate relations with my wife, but the pleasure remains just as high!

Chapter 7

Lower Back Pain, Surgeries, and Pain Management or An Israelite's Perspective of Wandering in the Wilderness for Forty Years

When it comes to the history of my back, I am not quite sure where to begin. Perhaps it is easier to say that I'm not sure where to end since the saga of back problems has continued now for over six years. I think that at this point it is sort of a question of what came first—the chicken or the egg? Or in my case, what comes first, the doctor or the pain? Since every time I see the doctor, my symptoms expand and my pain level increases. So, here I am after four surgeries over a six-year period—back to the beginning. I guess you could say that I am caught in some sort of time warp like Back to the Future, but instead of traveling in a DeLorean with Doc Brown, I seem to be tumbling through some sort of HMO worm hole with a variety of doctors that would most certainly fail a Stephen Spielberg screen test—even if they were trying out for the part of Jaws (the shark) or Jabba the Hut.

My challenge in the purpose of writing this book is to add some humor to my situation, and so I will do my best to deal with my back history—as baffling and frustrating and discouraging as it has been—in a way that will hopefully inspire others who may share similar health problems as my own, and learn as I have, to keep a smile on my face, at least while I share the tale of my back. I guess you might say that this could be considered a case of the tale wagging the back!

I can't be sure when my back problems actually began. I did not suffer a serious car accident or a bad fall at work. All I can say for certain is that the problems began to intensify as I reached the wonderful age of 45. I can also add that chronic back pain does run in the family. My dad had a deteriorating spine along with several surgeries. I can also say that at 6'5" tall, and weighing over 285 pounds, and with a pant inseam of 33 inches which means that I have a large upper torso, I was sort of destined to have back problems as I got older. I can also say that I further escalated my potential for back problems by doing stupid things. For example, for years, I used to love to go jogging. Now if someone out there has a similar build to mine, I would strongly suggest that you stop jogging, unless you are doing it on a very cushiony treadmill and start swimming. All of my doctors throughout this ordeal have come up with a myriad of theories as to the causes of my lower back pain. But, they have all concurred with this one bit of advice and so I will pass it on. If you are a larger person, you will be much better off if you swim for exercise rather than jog. You still get a very good cardiovascular workout, but with zero friction on your lower joints including knees and lower back. However, since I found out after the fact, I feel similar to the sexually active teen female that finds out about contraceptives after months of unprotected expressions of sexual freedom. By the time I had been counseled to swim instead of run, I too had already become impregnated and started to show signs of bulging—only my bulging was occurring in the discs of my lower spine.

Besides the jogging, I also loved the lower back pounding and knee-jolting fun that comes from "older guys" getting together at the local gym or fitness center to blow off some excessive testosterone as well as some much-needed joint tissue and bone fragments to play some basketball to show that they still got game. For years, you could find me down at the local gym's basketball court mingling with a group of older guys in pick-up games. If you have never watched a group of so called "grown up" men playing in such a situation, you are missing out on some great entertainment, and the best part is that it is free! Spectating at such an event really combines the best of many professional sports, all in the comfort and convenience and price range that everyone can enjoy.

Since we now find ourselves in some economic challenges where we have all had to tighten our financial belts a bit, I feel good as a fellow citizen by sharing with you a wonderful form of untapped entertainment that is very entertaining and free of charge (if you can ask the minimum wage-paid person sitting at the front desk of a fitness center loving their job as they advertise themselves to countless potential dating partners constantly walking through the front doors to let you in as you just want to watch the basketball pick-up game going on at center court). What other sporting event combines evidence and traces of an organized basketball game along with some football acquired skills including tackling, pushing, shoving, and profane expletives, added to the sweaty physical contact and verbal antagonizing of professional wrestling and the daring fashion trends of combining seldom-washed, sweat-stained and many times too revealing, once well-fitting but now stretched out shorts and T-shirts or tank tops that at some past time and place fi t well but are now bulging with masses of blubbery fl ab just screaming to break free from the fabric that was never intended to receive such tinsel-strength testing? What more could you ask for in an ultimate sporting experience—all free of charge?! So the next time you are looking for some great entertainment—including an out of the ordinary date idea, and you don't have any money, you know what to do. Perhaps if it catches on enough, we could make it into another great American pastime!

And so, in summary, I was born with a bad back, I have the stature of a back pain sufferer, and I participated in some athletic activities that I shouldn't have. Then, I turned 45 years old and the beast was unleashed!

I first realized I had a problem when I began to experience what is commonly referred to as my back began "going out" on me quite frequently. I'm not sure who originally came up with this phrase of a back "going out" on you. Although I use the phrase frequently and I hear others using it frequently, I do not think that it adequately describes what actually happens or what you actually feel during the experience. After all, the term "going out" usually refers to a date or an outing or an outdoor activity. So as far as the back is concerned, this just doesn't work as an explanation. However, if the term "going out" refers to someone who walks out the door to catch some fresh air only to find that the door is located at the edge of a cliff overhanging an endless dark abyss that one falls into and remains in a free fall state until the hole opens up into the inextinguishable flames of hell itself, then in that particular case, "going out" does adequately explain what actually occurs.

Originally, I thought that these episodes when my back "went out" were normal as I knew quite a few people who suffered from occasional back pain. And so, whenever I felt that twinge in my lower back from bending wrong or working out too hard or getting hammered by some Kobe Bryant wannabe in one of those basketball pick-up games, I would go to my regular doctor if I could get an appointment the same day as the incident—yeah right! The odds of that happening were about the same as getting a Playboy Mansion Sunday Brunch invitation from Hugh himself! Most likely, I would go to Urgent Care or the Emergency Room so that I could get some relief more quickly. (Relief referring to pain killers and muscle relaxers, which by the way, are almost as appealing as the brunch invite from Hef when you are in so much pain and discomfort! Then I would go home and lay down and take the pills and wake up about three days later feeling much better and longing for a few more pills to take the edge off. Little did I realize at the time that this little edge I was getting off of would erode into what would ultimately be compared to a drop off like the pit in the movie 300 where the Persian emissaries were mercilessly kicked off the ledge into a seemingly endless drop-off of certain doom by the Spartans who would not give in to the tyrannical demands of the self-proclaimed God-king Xeroxes.) Otherwise, I would have to be in a real bad state of pain to ever muster up the courage to enter the emergency room at the local hospital. I am not sure how many of you have been to a hospital emergency room before, but it is one place that makes me very concerned that if I were to survive the treatment I were to receive for my condition that I entered with, I would most surely die from some sort of illness or contagion I contracted from being exposed to a myriad of diseases, sickness, and illnesses carried by the odd sort of people in the emergency room waiting area. That emergency room waiting area is one of the few places on earth I have ever visited where my doubts of the earthly existence of extra-terrestrial beings have been deeply shaken to the very core of rational thought. This is one of only a very few places where I have seen such strange creatures speaking so many odd alien-type dialects and making such unearthly guttural and primeval sounds, as to make me look around to see if I am really in the hospital or if I am an extra in the filming of Men in Black 3!

Anyway, when I found myself in a great deal of back pain, I would seek out remedies to deal with the pain and receive the medical treatment needed to get back to my regular daily schedule. Unfortunately, the frequency and intensity of my back pain became so frequent that finally, I sought out medical advice on my alternatives for a more permanent cure of my constant problems.

My first referral was to a pain specialist who after several nerve functioning tests, x-rays, and an MRI, recommended that I receive a new procedure shown to be effective on almost 70% of all participants in a recent clinical study, known as the IDET procedure. This procedure was explained to me in a way that made sense. The doctor explained that when a bulging disc occurs, the disc protrudes out of the spinal column and can put pressure on the nerve that runs inside the nerve canal right next to the spinal vertebrae. When this happens, a patient has several choices. He can have a disc replacement surgery, or he can have the bulging part of the disc shaved off, or he could have his vertebrae fused together, or he can have a less evasive IDET procedure where a hot probe is inserted into the disc and the disc is heated up. The theory being that once the disc is heated, it will be malleable enough to reshape itself back into its original form contained within the vertebrae where it will no longer bulge and place pressure on the nerve. This made sense to me and so I authorized the procedure. Unfortunately, my case wasn't the same as the 70% in the study and resulting in no improvement. I later found out two things from the surgeon who fused my back. First, if the IDET doctor would have read the MRI correctly and not have been hungry for the fees collected as a result of this worthless procedure, he would have known that the results would have been ineffective because my main problem was not the shape of the disc, rather, it was the fact that I had very little disc left and the bone structure of my spine was all messed up. Second, my surgeon informed me that if an IDET procedure doesn't work, the result would be certain stiffening of the disc, causing it to be brittle and resulting in a 100% chance of disc replacement down the road if it didn't work. My surgeon also informed me that the MRI showed that I never had enough disc to work with to begin with, so that the results of the procedure were destined to be ineffective. Of course, the IDET doctor didn't inform me of that small detail that perhaps would have changed my original decision to go along with the IDET. By the way, when I was informed of this fact, I finally realized what the acronym IDET stands for: It means, "Idiot Doctor's Erroneous Treatment." If you conclude that the results of the procedure were as effective as the meaning behind the acronym, then you are correct in assuming that the treatment was absolutely worthless—except that now what was left of my disc would become brittle and begin to disintegrate rapidly.

The next phase of my back saga was to go and see a pain specialist. Of course, I had to wait and wait and wait for the authorizations to be approved from my primary care provider to go and see a so-called "pain specialist." I am not sure where this guy went to medical school, but I think that if you were to examine his diploma carefully, you would see fl ames, a pitchfork, a skull with crossbones, and a signature by the dean of the school—Lucifer, Son of Darkness. This guy's bedside manner was quite disturbing. He was mean, insensitive, and he treated me like some kind of heroin addict seeking relief from one of his infected needles of liquid death.

I don't know how many of you can relate a visit to your local doctor as being treated like a common criminal, a drug addict, or some kind of child-molesting serial killer. But as far as my history goes, I think that some doctors should enroll in more of the Patch Adams Philosophy of humane and sensitive treatment of patients, rather than The Grim Reaper's Deathbed Interview Tactics of Anxiety, Frustration and Terrorizing of the innocent, premium and co-paying patients. The other thing that really bothers me about HMO's is that many of them appear to have the philosophy to always take the path of least cost to get the end result—no matter how long and twisted that path is, or how many temporary fi x stops you take along the way—which will probably end up costing more than if they were to do it right the first time anyway! It appears that the desired end result of saving a few dollars is either premature and unnecessary death, or irreparable brain damage resulting in a patient ending up in some padded room somewhere in a strait jacket eating insect horsd' oeuvres. I realize this generalization could be considered unfair or over-generalizing, but I know too many people who have jumped through many fiery hoops like I have to get the proper treatment needed to actually be healed, while getting burned in the process.

After my pain specialist's intense interrogations that questioned whether or not I was really in pain, or just there as a ruse to satisfy my uncontrollable drug habit, he decided to give me a series of saddle blocks like an epidural that are designed to block the pain signal from my back to the pain center of my brain. And so, I received a series of three shots over a three-month period of time. Now I will admit that although these shots did work, they only lasted for a couple of weeks each time. As a result, the temporary relief of the shots did not do anything towards my back-healing process as the time bomb of my deteriorating spine continued to count down, and my condition worsened.

131

I now entered the next phase of treatment that I will refer to as the Pontius Pilate philosophy of the washing of hands to avoid the risk of actually liberating my condition of pain and suffering.

My HMO began a lengthy process of acquiring an MRI, which had to be repeated after several visits to two different neurologists who couldn't read the MRI because it was blurry. The first of these doctors said that my discs were deteriorating and there was nothing that could be done for me other than recommend a long-term, or life-long term of pain management, or in other words, pain killers and drooling in a recliner watching re-runs that I could not remember watching in the first place because I was stoned on opiates. The second neurologist, considered by some to be a pioneer in disc replacement surgery, told me that the procedure was too new and because I needed to replace two discs, he recommended that I wait two to three years to see how the long-term study results were turning out, and then to come back and see him for possible treatment at that time. These useless events took place over about a year and a half period of continually visiting my primary care physician and begging to see doctor after doctor after doctor.

Even through all the frustration and setbacks by doctors who would not or maybe could not help me, I remained optimistic that all I had to do was to find the right doctor. After all, I was in my forties, I was in pretty good shape and athletic, and I led a very active lifestyle even though I spent many days icing my back in my easy chair or on my bed.

During this challenging time in my life, I was inspired to stay positive and keep on living life on my terms. There were several key individuals that were the source of my inspiration. The most important person that has remained faithfully by my side through all the adversity and enduring all of my little attitude farts was my incredible wife. She has and always will be the single most motivational person in my life. She has stood by my pouting, my pain, my self-pity, my self-centered need for attention and care, and all of the other crap I dished out to her with a smile, an encouraging word, and a loving gesture. I cannot express in words the love and respect that I have for my wife—even though I don't always show it and I know that she deserves so much better. She truly is my angel sent from God. And, I freely admit that if I were to lose everything in my life—my health, my job, my home, my wealth (what little there is of it), and all of my earthly possessions, I would never have the justification to complain to God because He sent me my wife. She means everything, and she is everything to me!

The next sources of strength to me are my children. They are just the greatest! They bring me so much joy and happiness. They, which includes spouses with three of our four children, really do complete my wife and I. I was not the best parent in the world, but I do love my kids more than life itself, and they are the reason why I desire to live a long and full life. I want to share their experiences as they become parents, enter the work force, and begin their own families. I want to be a big part of that. And, I have made a promise to my kids that I will be around for a long time to see their kids grow up and share in my grandkids' lives as well. If I have any say in the matter, and I believe that I do through the life I lead and the decisions I make to stick around, I am going to stick around for a long time! And so, I am extremely motivated to keep on plugging away by staying busy and occupied with my time, as well as trying my best to deal with adversity through my expressions of humor.

I guess that my prescription for true happiness as a doctor with a degree in life is simply this: 1. Be close to your family and keep your family relationships the top priority in your life. 2. Acknowledge that there is a Supreme force or being or however you wish to express divine intervention in your life in some way and stay true to those beliefs in the way that you live and treat others. Finally, 3. When adversity hits, and it will hit believe you me, the best way to deal with adversity is with a spoonful of humor, or sugar as Mary Poppins would have said.

Besides my family relationships and several key friends and mentors I have had throughout my life, I must give special recognition to two other individuals that I became acquainted with during my time of physical and psychological challenges. One of these people is a man whom I met only once in a very random, casual situation. The other is a previous student of mine who remains a dear friend to this day. Both of these individuals reminded me that although I have my challenges— as we all do— there are others who have to deal with so much more adversity than we could ever imagine who make us feel so ridiculously selfish for even thinking to complain. When I think of these two individuals, I am reminded of a story that I heard once about a man who complained about needing new shoes until he saw a young boy who had no feet.

The first person is someone whose name I do not know. He also uses a wheel chair to get around. I bought peanuts from him one day while I was driving home after a long day of work when I found myself drowning in self-pity for all of my woes in life. The second person is a very dear friend of mine who has been a great source of strength and inspiration throughout my life. His name is Josh. Josh was a young man born with muscular dystrophy. He has been in a wheel chair since birth. He has had over 28 surgical procedures in his young 25 years of life. Currently, he is going to college and getting a degree in broadcasting while announcing the basketball games for the men's college team where he goes to school. He is a motivational speaker, he is my hero, and I am so honored and privileged to call him my friend.

I do not consider myself a professional poet, although I do enjoying writing. I do not attempt to write much poetry—except for the occasional holiday or birthday card. But in the case of these two individuals, I did write a poem about the inspirational influence each of them had on my life. I feel that at this point of my story, I should share these poems with you so that you can understand the impact these two individuals had on my life and how they have motivated me to overcome challenges, in the hopes of giving you some motivation and peace of mind as well.

The first poem is called "The Peanut Salesman."

The day had been long, my work was sure tough,
My head started to throb, the traffic was rough, As
the twilight set in, I turned on my lights, And
honked at the guy cutting in from the right.

The concourse of lights creeping along just ahead
Slipped me into a trance and my thoughts all led To
the injustices of God and the frustrations of life That
seemed to pierce my troubled soul like a knife.

My bills pile up high, the kids lack respect,
Both cars need repair, our weathered house shows neglect.
The garage is a mess! Our vacation fell through! I'd
like to go fishing, there's so much to do!

My knee has arthritis, my wife has the flu, My
hair's getting gray, my waistline sure grew. They
need volunteers at church and at school, I really
could help, but I'm sure no fool!

As I think of the future, I sink into my seat.
I'm so depressed now, I give in to defeat.
So, I pull off the road to get something to eat.
"Why not?" I say as I order a treat.
I parked the car in the lot on the side, to
get my food ready to eat for the ride.
As I pulled out to go, I noticed at the stop,
A man in a wheelchair, with a sign atop
Saying, "Peanuts For Sale, 5 bags for 2 dollars Or
12 bags for 5 dollars, if any prefers."
I pretend to ignore the man in the chair, And I
pulled out to go, leaving him there. I drove
about a block, then suddenly turned To go
back, though why I cannot discern.
I parked in a space close to his display And I
walked up to him, "Hello!" I say. I reached
out my hand to take his in mine, his eyes had
a twinkle, his smile was divine
His trembling hand remained at his side, He
could not move, but it looked like he tried.
He returned a big grin, and attempted to speak, But
the words never came, his voice was too weak.
His head strained to the side as he looked up at me
And a recording began from a speaker at his knee
Saying, "Twelve bags for five, or five bags for two
And for any business you give, I sincerely thank you!"
I placed a five in his pocket near his hand at his side
He acknowledged the act with a shaky nod of his head Then I
patted his shoulder, looked at him and said,
"Thank you, dear friend, the nuts I will love,
But you example to me is a sign from above

That where much is given, much is required."
"From this moment on, I will never grow tired of
facing adversity and life's little tests for you have
shown me that I am so blessed!"
I waved as I drove past my friend on the street Rolled
up my window, wiped a tear from my cheek.
I sang as I drove, the trip went by fast.
I soon arrived home and entered at last!
I rushed to my wife and gave her a big kiss
And hugged each of my children, not one did I miss. I
vowed to change my life's outlook that day
Because of the friend I chanced to meet on the way.

The second poem is about my friend Josh. I have coached basketball and football at the high school level for many years and Josh was our basketball and football team manager and basketball announcer for several years, as well as a student in my class and a dear friend. Our friendship and the strength of our relationship which was solidified through our experience in high school sports is analogized in this poem entitled, "The Hero of the Game"

If only I made that free throw,
If I hit just one more three,
If I wouldn't have missed that board,
If I just played better "D,"
Then I wouldn't drop my head in shame 'cause
I'd be the hero of the game.
If the refs didn't make that call,
If my leg wasn't so sore,
If my teammates would pass the ball,
If a decent crowd would ever show,
Then I'd make myself a name 'cause
I'd be the hero of the game.

If coach would call a better play,
If my shoes weren't so old, If that
noisy fan would go away, If I
didn't have this darn cold.
Then I'd build up quite the fame 'cause
I'd be the hero of the game.
There will always be another excuse
That someone as great as me can use To point
anywhere else the finger of blame To justify why I'll
never be the hero of the game.
I'd make that free throw!
I'd nail that three!
I'd get that board!
I'd shut 'em down with "D!" 'cause in my wheelchair, I
feel no shame when in my dreams, I'm happy just to
play the game.
I wouldn't mind the ref's call; I could handle
my legs being sore. I would pass my teammates
the ball, I would appreciate any fan to show.
'cause if I could just walk and not be lame, then
I'd be so honored just to play the game.
I would run any of coach's plays,
I wouldn't mind playing in shoes that are old.
I don't care if that noisy fan stays, I
can play through this little cold.
"Cause if just for a moment, God could straighten my frame,
my ultimate dream would come true—to just play in the game.
If we ever think to give an excuse
When we reflect on the talents God gave us to use,
the only man worthy to point a finger of shame Is my
friend Josh, the real hero of the game!

Okay, before we get carried away with the emotions, let's refocus on the story as this writing is supposed to stay on the lighter side. I will just say that the above relationships are real and these individuals have had and continue to have a significant impact on my life and how I deal with challenges in my life.

After the shots, I was finally referred to a neurologist/spinal surgeon. I have a great deal of faith in this doctor to this day. As of this writing, I am still seeing him for continued spinal problems. Before I saw him, I met with his partner who is a spinal diagnostics specialist. This doctor examined my MRI and determined that I have four bad discs, with the two lowest discs—L-5, S-1, and L-4 being the worst and needing treatment. (I think that is what they are referred to as I get a bit confused with all the number and letter combinations. Remember that I am a teacher and in education, we have so many acronyms for everything, I start to get a bit dyslexic when numbers and letters and abbreviations are put together.) You know how sometimes first impressions can be inaccurate? In my psychology class while discussing human behavior, we talk about the concept of judging others based upon our past experience. Well, as I entered the surgeon's office and saw his dreadlocks, I was momentarily taken off guard as this doctor's image didn't fi t any of my past experience. I guess that it would be sort of like going to a job interview for a position with a profession of distinction, only to sit down in the interview office and looking at the interviewer as he/she enters the office and finding this person of authority, experience, and wisdom to be Goofy from Disney animation fame! Once I sat down, my doctor started to interview me and show me the MRI while showing me the actual degeneration of the disc and explaining the condition of my discs and why they were causing me so much pain. Then, he took out a plastic model of a lower spine and he showed me all the components of the spine and their functions and how the symptoms, or the pain is generated from different sources based upon my actual condition. As he did so, the delusional loppy ears morphed back into his dreads, and the ridiculous canine smile disappeared into an expression of confidence and experience as my prejudgment radically transformed his image in my mind to a much broader picture of what a competent doctor looks like. And by the way, the pendulum of the image of what a good doctor actually looks like continues to swing back and forth to this day, as I continue to visit all kinds of doctors that are always redefining my preconceived notion of what a good doctor should or shouldn't look like.

Doctor dreadlocks seems to be a very competent neurologist, and even though I have recently requested a second opinion as my symptoms continue to cause me problems, I have maintained confidence in this doctor up until the present time, when after nine and a half months since his last outpatient procedure, I have had post-surgery symptoms including skin rashes, hot spots, skin discoloration, tissue swelling, nerve pain down both legs, a throbbing pain in the lower back region, and sensitivity to the touch in the area of the sutures where it feels like I just had the surgery and it hasn't healed yet. And so, after nine and a half months of visiting and revisiting him to discuss all of these symptoms, and having him review my recent MRI, he has had to refer me onto another series of specialists to deal with my unique set of symptoms, not directly related to my spine and nerve structure. I am now being told that I have what appears to be an autonomic nervous vascular disorder. I guess that at this point, Paul Harvey will just have to wait for "the rest of the story," as I have decided to move on with my life and stop living day to day, waiting for my primary health care provider to authorize my next set of referrals.

When it comes to getting good treatment from doctors, I have finally and painfully come to the conclusion that the challenge in finding the right doctor is this: you have to find the doctor who is best suited to treat your specific problems— and I really do mean very specific! For example, if you want to go out and eat real good Italian food, you don't go to a Chinese restaurant. If you want to eat a good steak, you don't go to a seafood place. So, when you want to get proper medical treatment, you have to find the very best doctor that is successful and has a very good reputation at treating the very specific symptoms that you have. At this point in my life, I'm afraid that my cravings for a good pizza have been substituted on my medical menu by some bad sushi!

I guess that I am getting ahead of myself in the story. Let's get back to where I was in the consultation stage with doctor dreadlocks. In the process of meeting with me over a series of visits, doctor dreads also consulted with his office partner who seldom performs surgery. This doctor is a neurologist who specializes in analyzing X-rays and MRI's and interpreting the condition of the spine and the best course of action to correct the problem and alleviate the pain caused by the deterioration of the spine and structures surrounding the nerves. I met with both of them separately and together, and they both recommended that I get a lower back fusion. The way I was explained this procedure is that they go in from the stomach. Then, they assess the condition of the discs and if they are bad, they replace the bad discs with a synthetic disc in between vertebrae. They then use three titanium screws to secure a titanium plate in front of the new artificial discs to keep them in place (since the spine bends forward and the discs could pop out if there were no plate to hold the discs in place).

That is what they ended up doing with me. So, off I went to a local hospital to get some metal surgically implanted titanium hardware in my back.

I don't remember anything about the usual prep work except for getting the good old IV, putting on the always too small gown that slides up my lower body and ends up to looking like Ellie Mae's tied off, midriff exposing blouse. The only differences between me and Ellie Mae is that for one, she has pants on while I have nothing on, and two, Ellie Mae looks a heck of a lot better in a blouse than I do! I always remember being gourneyed into the operating room. Then, they helped me onto the operating table with all of the lights and sterile stainless-steel instruments and computer screens and the music playing. Next, came one more quick little interview with the anesthesiologist making sure that I am not allergic to anything and explaining to me that he was about to give me a sedative through the IV that would put me to sleeeeeee.......p.

Then the next thing I know, I am fighting to stay awake, I am in and out of consciousness, and my back hurts like hell! I find myself in the worst episode of The Twilight Zone ever imagined. Or in other words, I am now in the recovery room! I imagine that recovery after a general anesthetic surgery must be similar to coming off a bad trip from a very addictive hallucinogenic. I was in and out of consciousness, begging for more morphine, and in a lot of pain. I remember wanting to get out of there, except that I liked the fact that a nurse was constantly by my side asking me if I needed more morphine and some ice chips. I kept fading in and out of consciousness with my brain trying to focus but unable to do so. I now know what an infant feels like when his "cute" mom holds his bottle just out of reach thinking that her infant can somehow take charge of his underdeveloped eye-hand coordination and motor skills and miraculously reach out and grab the bottle with total control. In fact, in re-visualizing this experience, I have just created a false memory of childhood that never actually happened to me—and while holding that newly etched memory as an infant, I just mentally babbled the sound "she-she mama dada baba," which interpreted means, "crap mom, give me that damn bottle!" I will never forget this traumatic experience that has been repressed in my subconscious mind and now resurfaced through the psycho-therapeutic writing of these memoirs.

I really do not remember my doctor coming to see me in recovery. My memories of recovery are real hazy—like having a weird dream in the middle of the night only to wake up the next morning with only the memory that you had a dream, but not remembering what it was about. However, I do know that my surgeon came in to see me and my wife to summarize the procedure and to reassure me that he had left specific instructions with the nursing staff to give me maximum doses of morphine once I left recovery and went to my room. Then, he was off to perform his next surgery. I know that the poor guy performs on average four procedures on his surgery days and they can last up to four hours each. I must say that I do feel bad for the doctors who are governed by the HMO's who dictate to them when they can operate and how much they can charge. I wonder what will happen if our medical care ever becomes nationalized and the government decides who will provide the care and what they can charge. The very thought of this makes me a bit queasy to say the least! Enough of the politics. This bit of evidence that my surgeon told us about his making sure with the nurses that my pain would be taken care of seemed like standard operating procedure at the time, but it will become critical in the story as it unfolds.

After spending several hours in recovery and dining on my post-op liquid diet of morphine injections and ice chips, I was wheeled up to my private room for some peace and quiet. Oh, wait a minute, all the rooms were full and so they wheeled me down to the end of some hallway and stuck me in a storage room a long way away from any nurse's station and not anywhere near an air conditioning duct. And, my nearest roommate I could detect was some woman located somewhere down the hallway, who based on the symptoms I witnessed, must have been suffering from anxiety and Alzheimer's. So, there I was; I had stripped down to just a washcloth covering my private area like a loincloth, and still sweating from the trauma and the heat. I was in terrible pain, and my wife had gone out to make cell phone calls to a few family members and friends to tell them the "good news" reported to her by the doctor while I was in my semi-conscious stupor in the recovery room. I was hot and sweating, and my pain meds were starting to wear off. What was worse is that my roommate down the hall kept crying out for help. In any other situation, I would have been very sad for this woman. She was obviously upset. She didn't know where she was, she wanted to go home, and she was surrounded by hospital staff and strangers whom she didn't recognize. But, every time I yelled out for help, begging for some medication and some air conditioning, my voice was drowned out by this woman whose room was located somewhere between the nurse's station and me. I admit that at the time, I wasn't in a rational state of mind as I continued to yell for some help while the woman was screaming for her own assistance. We must have sounded like some musical duet gone terribly wrong. If this were an audition for American Idol, I doubt that even Paula could have found something nice to say about our little number! But, I was in a lot of pain and getting desperate with the thought that I was being neglected. So, I kept on screaming for help and the nurses continued to ignore us both.

Finally, my wife found my storage room and entered with her good friend. As they entered, the situation before them must have appeared to be somewhat comical, but they had the wisdom to hold back any sort of smile, let alone any laughter. The corners of both of their mouths twitched ever so quickly. I could see both of them biting their tongues. They both knew that any sort of humorous response would not be appropriate. It was very obvious that I was very uncomfortable. Knowing that I was in obvious need, they wisely did not ask if I needed anything. That type of question in this situation reminds me of a book I once read that was entitled, "Witty Comebacks for Stupid Questions," or something like that. The inspiration from this book came from a frequent segment out of Mad Magazine, if I recall the source correctly. This book had some very quick responses as a result of some idiot lacking common sense asking a question so obvious that it was borderline material for the severely mentally challenged. An example from this book would show an illustration of a guy in a suit walking down a remote dusty road out in the middle of nowhere with a gas can in his hand, being followed by several lizards with canteens and umbrellas. The guy's tongue would be hanging halfway down his body covered with big balls of cotton. His necktie would be wrapped around his head like Rambo's headband. His cracked and bleeding toes would be sticking out of his disintegrated shoes, and he would be crawling on all fours, looking like his next move would be to keel over in death by dehydration. And, while he is looking up at the service station attendant whose intellectual appearance would have made Gomer Pyle look like a Princeton scholar and the banjo player in "Deliverance appear to be an MIT graduate, the attendant asks, "Did you run out of gas?" Then the classy comeback of the guy to the attendant would be something like this, "No, I didn't run out of gas, I just wanted to take a break from my boring drive and walk all this way to have a stimulating conversation with a genius like you!" Or, "No, I didn't run out of gas, I am actually a gas can salesman and I was wondering if you would like to buy

this one at a great price as it is my last display model."

Instead, my wife's friend who really is a take charge person asked me what I needed with the reassurance and conviction in her voice that indicated to me that she would get it done and quick. Before I give you my response here I must say that I really am not a person who cusses that much. My wife never cusses nor does this friend of ours. And under normal circumstances, if I were to cuss in front of them, I would embarrass my wife and offend her friend. However, these were anything but normal circumstances. I was recovering from (up to that point) the most extensive surgery of my life, I was in a great deal of pain, my nurses were nowhere to be found, it was very hot, and there was a screaming lunatic down the hall. And so yes, I did blurt out a few cuss words as I told these two very proper ladies that I was in a great deal of (bleep) pain, I needed some (bleep) pain medication now, and I was very (bleep) hot and uncomfortable and I (bleep) needed a (bleep) room with (bleep) air conditioning or at least a (bleep) damp, (bleep) cool (bleep) wash (bleepity-bleepin' bleep) cloth. Wow, that was bleeping therapeutic!

I will mention here that I did notice there was a tube going down the middle of my bed and attached to a bag at the foot of the bed. I realized that this was a catheter. The medical staff had the good sense and probably a premonition to plant the device while I was under anesthetic. I really didn't notice it that much anyway since I was pretty sedated.

With my motivating speech, my wife and her friend both took immediate action. First, they went and got the nurse. When the nurse got there, she demonstrated that she had not read my book by asking if I needed something for the pain. Instinctively, I glanced around the room to see if I could find the lizards or the banjo. No luck! I told her that I was in extreme pain and that I needed some relief. My wife informed the nurse that my surgeon had confirmed to her that he had left explicit instructions to give me whatever I needed to make sure that I was comfortable. The nurse said that she would try to contact the doctor to increase the dosage. My wife told the nurse that the doctor was in surgery and that he had left word to give me maximum pain medication. The nurse said that it was against hospital procedure to give me any more pain medication without confirmation from the doctor. I squinted my eyes in focusing in on the nurse's nametag. It seems that I remember her name looked like or reminded me of "Satan." Since many names have a masculine and a feminine version, I wonder if there is such a thing as Satania or Luciferia. If there is, that was her name for sure.

The next thing that happened is that I had a déjà vu moment in the form of a flashback of my book as she asked her second real intelligent question, which was "Are you hot?" I felt like making up an answer that would or sure be included in the second book entitled, "More Witty Comebacks to Stupid Questions" like, "No I'm not hot, I actually strip down butt naked and sweat profusely whenever I am really cold. It's my body's way of faking me out whenever I get too cold!" Even if she never read the book, I think that she caught the sarcasm in my voice. Or perhaps, she got the idea when she noticed my trembling hands reaching upward in a vain attempt to wrap them around her neck and squeeze her neck until her head popped off. My wife suggested that if I could get another washcloth (since the first one was occupied) and some ice, she would put the ice in the washcloth and cool off my forehead. Luciferia smiled and went on her way to try to contact my doctor and get the ice and washcloth. I guess she figured that filling one out of two requests was acceptable. I did get some ice chips and the washcloth, and she even brought me an additional cup of ice chips to replenish some of my body fluids that were drenching my bedding.

I am not sure how long I had to wait for the nurse to get the approval for more medication, but as soon as my surgeon finished his next surgery, he checked his pager and found out that I was requesting more medication. I guess that he has some pull around the hospital because he came by to see how I was doing and when he found out how much pain I was in, he excused himself and took a brisk walk down the hallway. Five minutes later, the nurse was at my bedside with a huge apology and a most wonderful machine called a morphine drip. I smiled uninhibitedly directly up into the face of the beast—uh I mean Satania—er, uh, the nurse I mean. This magnificent device was hooked up to my IV and it came with a hand-held push button so that every eight minutes, I could push the button and the machine's pump would activate sending the morphine nectar of the pain gods down the tube and into my IV. I know for a definite fact that for the next 48 hours or so until I was sent home, I never missed an eight-minute interim for the juice. I am sure that as soon as the timing mechanism clicked over at the eight-minute mark and thus electronically authorizing the morphine hit, My thumb was depressing the button so that the two were as synchronized as the gold medal winning synchronized swim team. As a result of this experience, I was concerned that I had obsessive-compulsive disorder, as my thumb kept twitching uncontrollably every eight minutes for several months after the pump had been removed. But, just as Pavlov's dogs forgot to salivate after several weeks of not hearing the bell ring, my thumb finally stopped on its own without having to go through some behavior altering counter-conditioning psychotherapy. It also took me several months to return to my normal sleeping habits of sleeping uninterruptedly through the night without waking up every eight minutes with my thumb pressing down on my pillow.

I spent the next two days in the hallway, with my roommate down the hall to give me the reassurance that I was never truly alone, and my new handheld computer game called "Morphine Invasion" which I never ceased to play. I only wish that they let me take the game home along with a lifetime supply of game cartridges (morphine). I also had the opportunity to choose my daily meal selections from the good old hospital menu. I am really not sure how a person gets selected for the job of hospital chef. I believe that these chefs come from one of two sources. Either these people flunked out of every culinary class available through public and private vocational training which qualifies them for a successful career in hospital cuisine, or they suffer from anti-social personality disorder and this is some sort of behavioral modification program to simulate the feelings of being a sociopathic serial killer by creating meals that torture poor innocent helpless patients and thus give the chef a euphoric feeling similar to the torture of insects and small animals or the graduated need to dismember their human victims who unknowingly await their fate being tube-strapped to a hospital bed. This hypothesis is further reinforced by the fact that even though we do see a menu and we do give it to a nurse, we never see the actual hospital cafeteria staff, thus protecting their anonymity making it impossible for us to identify our suspect in some sort of line-up behind a two-way mirror looking into the kitchen. I have eaten enough hospital food to believe that if we were able to look into a two-way mirror showing the hospital chefs at work without knowing that we were watching, the scene would look something like demonic witches and warlocks with long, warted noses and yellow, crooked teeth and knarled up fingers standing around big cauldrons hideously cackling as they stirred in bat wings, eyes of newt, crow innards, and a host of other ingredients from Beelzebub's kitchen.

Finally, the two days were over and it was time to go home. The nurse came in and informed me that it was time to remove the catheter. Boy, that was a relief! She briefly reviewed the Lamaze method of controlled breathing in through my nose and out through my mouth that I would need to focus on as she pulled out the tube. And so, as I began my breathing exercise, she pulled out the tube.

This experience reminds me of being with my wife during the birth of our first child. Being new parents and all, we were encouraged to sign up for a Lamaze class offered by the hospital and so we did. After all, we wanted to do everything by the rules and we were confident that this was something that we needed to do for the benefit of the baby. We had seen Lamaze practiced by birthing experiences on television and movies and we felt confident that this method would ease the pain suffered by my wife during delivery—especially since the women on TV and the movies always breathed and their husbands were there to coach them on and it was not only an effective tool in pain control, but it was also a bonding experience for mother and father during this wonder event. What we didn't fully realize at the time was that Hollywood has a way of simplifying the procedure and making the moment of birth out to be quick and easy and not too painful. Yes, the mothers-to-be do scream, and the doctor does encourage them to push, and the husband is right there to wipe her brow with a cool, damp cloth and to lovingly encourage her to control her breathing. But in the movies, there are a few quick pushes, a bit of yelling, and then the next thing you know, the actor-doctor is handing a beautiful (2-month old stand in) baby to the mother neatly wrapped in a blanket and exclaiming, "It's a beautiful boy!" And the new mom and dad smile at each other with teary eyes and the husband gently kisses his wife on the forehead and the scene fades to black as the scene ends.

In our own experience, it did not go down quite like this. First of all, at six weeks before the scheduled full-term arrival, my wife's embryonic sack sprung a leak. I remember that she informed me that this had happened early in the morning of a workday. As she had not yet begun contractions, we didn't feel rushed to get to the hospital and so I called work to tell them that I would not be coming in that day. Since she was not in labor, we were in no hurry and so we lounged in bed and watched The Price is Right with Bob Barker. After the showcase showdown, we got dressed and headed down to the hospital. When we got there, we filled out all the admitting forms and my wife was checked in. We met with the doctor who told us that since the baby was early, they wanted to wait as long as possible but after three days, they would have to induce the labor since there was a chance for infection through the little leak. The doctors wanted to wait to allow the baby's lungs to develop since he was premature and once the embryonic sack opens, there is a response in the respiratory system of the fetus to get ready to start breathing on their own. (Sorry for the lack of medical terms, but I can't remember them all and they really aren't that important to the story since this is not an article for submission in some medical journal.) The doctors wanted my wife to stay in the hospital to keep her in a sterile environment to reduce the likelihood of infection and so we waited.

I remember that first night she was in the hospital, we were to go to our last birthing class. Well, since we were already at the hospital, I figured that I might as well go to the class as I felt a sudden urge to graduate with honors from a class that I was about to put into practice in a real-life situation. As I entered the class, I greeted the other couples and we all sat down. I remember the nurse running the class asking me where my wife was. I told her that her water had sprung a leak and that she was down in labor and delivery. I remember her asking me with quite a bit of intensity why I was in the class and not with my wife! I informed her that she was not in labor and that the doctors would not induce labor for another two days, so I thought I should show up to get any final instructions before the big event. Of course, congratulations were expressed to me by the other couples as we completed the final course where we were shown a video of an actual childbirth with the couple engaged in a very rigorous and disciplined breathing routine. I remember feeling confident that I could go into the delivery and motivate my partner to breathe together in a performance that would far surpass the breathing of the amateurs in the video. Little did I realize then that if our Lamaze experience were the final exam in our parenting class, we would both flunk the class!

Anyway, after the three days, the doctors were concerned that the possibility of infection outweighed the concern that our baby's lungs were fully developed and so my wife was given an IV solution that would induce her labor. We were informed that the medication would take 8 to 10 hours to take effect. They also informed us that induced labor typically made labor pains longer and more intense than in ordinary deliveries. (We both thought how friggin' great that tidbit of news was!)

The 72 hours passed by quickly and the labor and delivery nurse started the IV drip to induce my wife's labor. After several hours, she began to experience labor pains, and so I remained vigilant by her side to give her encouragement and to hold her hand during the contractions that began to come more rapidly and more intensely as time went on. I remember that my wife was in a lot of pain and yet her cervix had not dilated much—at least in the initial hours of the IV. In fact, it was only after about eight long and excruciatingly painful hours that she began to dilate, and by that time, she was not in a very good mood and the blame for all of the pain and discomfort began to be placed on my shoulders by my wife who was becoming more and more agitated in her speech. Of course my wife had long decided that she wanted to have an epidural, or a sort of spinal block shot to alleviate the intense pain she was experiencing. She had asked for it early on in her labor pains but the nurses wanted her to wait so that they could monitor her contractions and make sure that she was progressing to avoid any possible infection. They were also taking periodic blood work to make sure that the baby was safe from infection. I felt so bad for her! I could do nothing to relieve her pain and so I held her hand and tried to give her words of comfort. I tried kissing her gently on the cheek and caressing her hands and face to help her feel better, but the longer the labor lasted, the angrier my wife got with me. I figured the least I could do was to stay by her side and take the blame as best I could by agreeing with her that this was all my fault. Also, along the way, her sense of smell became much more acute than usual because all of a sudden, I started to smell bad to my wife, which agitated her further and made her more upset. All at once she would yell at me that I smelled and that her pain was my entire fault and to get away from her.

Then, just as I was honoring her request and began to leave the room, she would start to cry and tell me that she loved me and she would beg me to come back and hold her hand. This happened several times, and each time I would do whatever she asked whether it was to get the hell out of there or to come back and hold her hand. At one critical point, the memory of the Lamaze classes entered my mind and I thought that I could sit on the bedside and be her breathing coach. So, I sat on the edge of the bed and told her to breathe as I demonstrated the rapid breathing techniques of breathing out the mouth in short successive bursts of breathing. I tried several times, but each time I did the demonstration, she would just look into my eyes with the most disturbing, soul-penetrating glare I have ever seen and tell me to shut up and quit breathing because my breath smelled bad and I was just annoying her and making her pain worse. With the determination and tenderness of the husbands in the video, I persisted. But the results were always the same. I was rejected and sent away. And then, just at the point of total despair on my part as my wife was just about ready to eviscerate me with a scalpel, or any other object within reach, the nurse came in and told her that she could now have the epidural if she still wanted it. Of course, her response was yes and she was comforted with the news that the pain would soon go away. All they had to do was stick the needle into her lower spine and numb the pain from her waist down. The nurse made it sound so wonderful. I guess that this bit of news is sort of like being told that your name was just selected as a finalist in the Publisher's Clearing House Sweepstakes. But what they didn't tell you was that 10 million other names were also selected as finalists as well. Because in my wife's case, after three attempts at getting the needle in the right place and being told by the nurse that in fact the needle "this time" had found it's mark, she was still in extreme pain and the shot never took. By the time she asked for the fourth attempt, she had reached ten centimeters and she was now ready to deliver, having gone through ten hours of very hard and intense labor pains that had been magnified and intensified by inducing of her labor.

She was wheeled into the delivery room where they placed her quivering legs up into the stirrups and as the doctor arrived, he instructed her to push as each set of contractions hit. As I witnessed the pain and agony my wife was going through, I realized how deceitful Hollywood had been over the years by falsely reenacting what it would be like for a woman to crap a peanut rather than deliver a baby. My wife was nauseated, and I held the little barf tray as she would push and puke, all in the same motion. Finally, the baby crowned, and the doctor asked her to summon up enough strength to give a few more pushes to get the baby out. I know that my wife had done all she could when as the doctor instructed her to bear down and push again, she yelled back at him to get the forceps and grab our baby by the head with them and pull him out the rest of the way. She had absolutely had enough! He told her that he couldn't do that as the forceps could put a strain on the baby's head and he sort of chuckled as he thought she was joking. But he soon found out that she was completely serious, as she demanded again that he do the rest with the forceps, I guess kind of like serving a dinner salad to guests with salad tongs! I began to give my wife what I felt to be a rational explanation as to why s the doctor couldn't follow her request, but I was stopped in mid-sentence with one fi ery look from my wife's piercing eyes. After a bit of further gentle persuasion from the doctor, my wife complied with a few more pushes before the doctor helped with the salad tongs and our first-born son entered this world. What an awesome experience! He was purple and covered with cottage cheese, but he was beautiful, and I loved my wife at that moment more than I had ever loved her before.

I have said many times that if men were to be the ones to carry and deliver babies, mankind would most certainly become extinct. The amazing thing about women giving birth is that they approach death's doors through so much discomfort while carrying the baby and so much intense pain at delivery, and then after a resting period, many of them go through it all over again, and sometimes again, and sometimes again! That is amazing to me. Men would do it in a test tube, or in a surrogate carrier of some kind, or they would not do it at all!

The irony of my wife's epidural experience was that right after delivery, her right leg became completely numb. We found this out because after some rest, she had to go to the bathroom and as she put her feet down on the floor and went to stand up, her right leg totally gave out and she collapsed on the floor. The epidural had finally taken effect! Only it was several hours after the delivery and it lasted four or five days before she could actually walk on her own!

I guess that this experience didn't really compare too much to the removal of my catheter. In fact, comparing the pain and trauma of giving birth to the discomfort experienced from the insertion or removal of a catheter really is quite ridiculous.

However, it does make for a good story and it most certainly validates my belief that if men rather than women had the physiological make-up to give birth, then mankind would have become extinct thousands of years ago. As I reread this analogy to myself, I actually feel a bit embarrassed that I would be so bold as to make such a comparison as being similar. I want you to know that I am not delusional. I actually do realize that a catheter is only a tube—not a six to nine-pound life form. And I must confess that I am a complete wimp in admitting that the result from the removal of the tube from the male's reproductive part does cause a considerable amount of pain, anguish, and distress. All I can really compare as similar between childbirth and the catheter is that the breathing methods taught by the medical staff is quite similar—although there is no such thing as a penis catheter insertion and removal class offered by the hospital before the event occurs. Because if there were, and guys saw the video before the actual event, they would never show up for the surgery and take their chances without medical help!

After spending the two days in the hospital and going through the agony and the ecstasy of parting with the catheter (ecstasy), and having to be detached from my wonderful morphine drip machine (agony), I was sent home to recover. I was in a very considerable amount of pain, but I was given a new friend to replace the old one who had to stay at the hospital (the drip). The name of this new friend was called Norco, and we soon became very close friends. In fact, we became almost inseparable! Just like Mary and her little lamb, everywhere I went, Norco was sure to go! I immediately became very fond of my new friend. You might even say that we bonded very quickly. Little did I know how strong this bond would become and how difficult it would be down the road to part ways when the time came. But for then, I was happy knowing that for the moment, no one could come between us. I soon found out that our relationship became very dependent upon that very concept—that our relationship became very schedule oriented — "one to two every four hours as needed for pain." Refer back to the beginning of chapter four if you forgot how attached my new friend and I had become. All I can say is that after a while, my friend and I began to abuse our relationship. He wanted more and more of my attention, and I needed and pleaded for more and more of his constant companionship. Fortunately, and in a very literal life-saving opportunity, I met with a very good pain management specialist who helped me break off the relationship and move on or should I say back up to realize the importance of the critical and valuable relationships that already filled my life—those of my wife and kids and family and dear friends.

My back started to get better and I continued to live smarter through improved eating habits and smart activities to maintain a healthier lifestyle by limiting my physical activities, without going overboard and risk a reinjury. For two years, I felt pretty good and my back was doing better. However, because of my degenerative condition and as a result of some developing bone spurs and scar tissue, some of the pain returned and I began to re-experience shots of nerve pain going down my leg and a throbbing pain that settled into my lower back region on an almost daily basis. Some days were worse than others, but when the good days began to disappear, and the bad days became my "normal" condition, I decided to go back to my primary doctor for treatment and to get a reauthorization to go and see my surgeon, Dr. Dreads, once again.

As I began the process of returning to see the doctor, I figured that it would be easy enough to go and see my surgeon again—especially since he was the one who had treated me and who was so familiar with my condition—WRONG! After my final follow-up visit with Dr. Dreads, his notes to my primary care physician said in effect that his work was now complete, and any further needs could be met through my primary care provider. So, when the pain returned, and I tried to set up an appointment with the surgeon again, his nurse told me that my primary care health provider denied the request. So, I had to start the process all over again. I went to my physician for several visits with little help. Over a period of several months of inquiry, we found out that my surgeon needed to submit an addendum to his original notes and send it to my provider's office to the person in charge of claims and referrals stating that if I had any further complications as a result of my pre-existing lower back conditions, I was to return back and see him for consultation and possible treatment. He did so and finally, I was allowed to go back and see my surgeon again.

I remembered at the time of my fusion the doctor told me that if I continued to have further problems with nerve pain, there was one more simple outpatient procedure that he could do to open up the nerve canal in my lower spine, and so when we met, I reminded him of that conversation of which he kept record. He felt that this procedure made a lot of sense as it should alleviate my pain and discomfort. So, we scheduled the outpatient procedure to be done during the month of August, so that I could convalesce before school started up again and not miss any work. The procedure took a couple of hours under general anesthetic. When it was finished and I came to, I was told that the nerve canal had successfully been cleaned out—along with some scar tissue that had accumulated around the nerve, and that now after all this time and all these procedures and treatment, my back should be in good shape. Little did I realize at the time that my problems were just beginning! The result of this procedure would lead me on a trek that would make Frodo Baggins' journey to rid middle earth of the ring seem like a walk in the park, a jog around the block, a sleigh ride over the river and through the woods to grandma's house, or any other little trip of small consequence.

It was a typically already hot, Inland Empire early morning in August in Southern California as I checked in to the outpatient surgical ward. I was to be one of the first procedures of the day. I went through the normal drill of changing into the cute little gown. Then I went to lay down on the always too small pre-op gurney where the nurse carefully placed the IV into my arm followed by two nurses and the anesthesiologist surveying me about possible complications or reactions or maiming, or even death that could possibly occur as a result of the anesthetic, while giving me the reassurance that it would not likely happen. Then, I signed my life away and released all hospital staff from the administrator down to the part-time custodian from any and all liability associated with either directly or indirectly or consequentially or otherwise, any complications as a result of the surgery. I will say in their behalf that I have always found the surgical nurses to be very professional and congenial, and some of them are actually quite hot. I don't know what it is about a woman in hospital uniforms— whether she wears pastels, cute animals or cartoon characters, or even in the good old hospital green. Or, maybe it is the fact that they could create in my subconscious mind some sort of savior complex. Or maybe these outfits are manufactured with some sort of pheromone that the uniform gives off that sends a hormonal signal straight to the arousal center of a male's brain. Whatever it is, and I do want my wife to know that I will always be faithful to her and love only her, there is just something about a woman in hospital fatigues that gets to me. Come to think of it, when my wife and I first got married, she worked in a dental office and she wore those cute little outfits! Perhaps some psychological researcher will take on this theory and test out the hypothesis to see if there is any evidence to support these subliminal powers of attraction that hold men completely defenseless as we place our lives in the care of nurses in uniform. Either that or I have just exposed myself to have some kind of kinky obsession for nurses!

When my turn came up, I was wheeled in to the chilly operating room where gloves and masks were donned, and some sort of quasi-Bob Marley music was playing in the background (perhaps the choice of my dreadlocked surgeon). I remember that the anesthesiologist started to say something about giving me something that was going to put me to sleeeeeee...zzzzzzzzp.

The next thing I knew, I was back in the recovery room talking to a hot nurse—oops, sorry—a professional health care worker— and I was a bit dizzy and nauseous. I remember the nurse giving me a shot for pain as she noticed my obvious discomfort. When she asked me if I needed anything, like some ice chips or some juice, I impulsively asked if I could get hooked up to a morphine drip machine. She laughed and so I smiled to go along with what she perceived as a joke and I settled for some juice. My surgeon came in and said that the surgery was a success. He widened the restricted nerve canal and he also removed some scar tissue that had built up in the area of my previous fusion. He told me that I was to call his office and set up a follow-up visit in three weeks and he exited to go and begin his second of I believe four procedures that day. My wife soon came in to join me and after several hours of recovery and my focusing all my attention to the conversation with my wife and not even glancing at any of the recovery room nurses—that is until one came over to review the post-op instructions of what to do and any trouble signs to look for once I returned home. Then I was wheeled out to the van and we drove home with a perceived reassurance that my back would finally be better, and I could return to somewhat of a normal lifestyle, provided that I used good judgment and common sense in my level and restrictions of daily physical activity.

This is where the chapter should end. But as my fate would have it, and if Paul Harvey were investigating this potential story of medical achievement, this is where he would begin "The rest of the story."

During the three weeks following the surgery, I was still in quite a bit of pain and I was "taking it easy" as far as my daily activity was concerned. But, as the follow up appointment with my surgeon approached, I was optimistic that the recovery would go as planned and I would be free from the bondage of chronic pain. (If you are or ever have been a sufferer of chronic pain, you would know exactly what I mean by using the word bondage.) We discussed my progress and we both felt good about the prognosis. I even felt so good that I had previously found out by listening in on one of the conversations between my surgeon and his office staff that he really only had two past times outside of his practice. One was golf, and the other was an occasional glass of good scotch. So on that particular visit, I wanted to do something to show my appreciation for my surgeon and his staff, who by the way I hold in very high regard, even though my particular road to recovery has been a difficult one with a few rockslides and fallen trees that have obstructed the way. So, I brought the staff a couple of cheesecakes and I brought my doctor a bottle of good scotch that just so happened to come with a couple of golf balls that had been branded with the logo of that particular brand of scotch. Now I must say that I do not drink. The reason should be quite obvious. I am sure that I was born with an addiction gene that if activated by certain behaviors or substances, would get out of control. My dad and mom had this gene, and so did several of my other close family members. So, before I went to purchase the scotch at a liquor store that prior to this point, I had frequented only to purchase a newspaper or an emergency gallon of milk as that is not my store of choice for milk, I had to find out what type of scotch my doctor preferred. So I called the doctor's office and asked one of the staff to find out for me. She did so and called back with the information. I was pleased with my idea to do something nice for my doctor and his staff as I left my home an hour early and purchased the cheese cakes and then continued my journey to a liquor store along the way.

Looking back on this decision to buy the scotch, I would have been much more financially better off today had I based my purchase on the premise of really nothing more than a token gesture of gratitude on a dozen name brand golf balls. For as the clock was ticking down to the scheduled time of my appointment, and I could not locate a liquor discount store, I was amazed as I went from grocery store to liquor store and priced scotch, that is was so expensive! Since I was told a particular brand of scotch, I was limiting my search to that particular brand. I was not going to buy some generic brand. That could not only come off as cheap, but also influence the quality of any future treatment. I remember finding one price label at a grocery store that looked very promising—until I read the fi ne print that showed the price was actually only the price per ounce! Finally, I was stuck with the very last liquor store by the doctor's office. Time had run out and I had to make my purchase. The store clerk was helpful, and I think he could see the word "CHEAPSKATE" etched on my forehead as he realized that I had limited funds. And even though I never mentioned golf balls to him as I was confident that there was not an impulse purchase rack of golf balls in the small liquor store (although there very well could have been based on what I know about golfers and drinking), he told me that he thought he had a bottle or two of the brand I was searching for that was being offered at a special promotion. He excused himself and returned a few minutes later with the bottle in a nice box that had two golf balls included in the price, and running out of time, I said. "I'll take it!" And in actuality, if you figure that each golf ball with the special logo attached cost me $10 per ball, then I got a real good deal on the scotch!

I made it to my appointment on time and the gifts were received with gracious gratitude. They all said that the gesture was very thoughtful but not necessary. NOW THAT I HAD TO GET A SECOND MORTGAGE ON MY HOME THEY TELL ME!

My surgeon's office is filled with some very nice, professional women who just coincidentally wear nurse fatigues. But, since my surgeon is the only male in the office, I thought it ironic and mentioned so to the doctor that along with the scotch, it was nice to have an extra set of balls around his office, because you just never knew when an extra set of balls would come in handy in an office full of women, etc. etc. etc. I guess that I milked that ball joke for as much mileage as I could get. After all, I did want to get some of my money's worth from my substantial investment!

The appointment overall went well, but there was some swelling and skin discoloration around the area of my lower back that was sutured. The doctor put me on some antibiotics and told me that the reason was most likely due to nothing more than one of the internal sutures had not yet dissolved. This did make sense to me as I do have allergic reactions to certain types of surgical bandage materials as I have already explained in the chapter on hernias. So, I left the office feeling good about my gifts and confident that the suture would dissolve, and the prescribed medicine would prevent any further infection. Yeah right!

This condition that appeared to be some kind of infection continued to grab my attention. It did not go away. At night, the incision area would get so hot that I would have to get up in the middle of the night and ice it to cool it down and be comfortable enough to get back to sleep. The swelling also continued to fill the surrounding tissue with fluids that placed pressure on my lower back nerves and made my lower back pain to intensify at times, to be even worse than before the surgery. So, I went back to see him and this time I just saw the nurse who changed the dressing and was advised to continue to take the antibiotics.

Over the next couple of weeks, the swelling, red skin and lower back pain intensified. And one evening during the third week, a heat rash formed on the area of skin just below the incision. This rash continued to get very hot, and at about midnight one night, several layers of skin started to peel off, leaving a very sensitive area of new skin beginning to develop—like the skin layer exposed after peeling from a real bad sunburn. This symptom scared me enough to go to the hospital emergency room as the urgent care facility had already closed. So, I drove down there to enjoy the ambiance of the

ER waiting room and treating area. This place is certainly like Forrest Gump's proverbial box of chocolates — "you never know what you are going to get" as far as who may be in the waiting room and what kind of curious or disturbing ailments they may have, or who was being treated back in the little curtained off rooms that were anything but private! After waiting for an hour or so, I was called back to see a doctor. He looked at the area and quickly had a nurse give me an IV while he scheduled a CT scan to check out the area. The IV bag, which contained a strong dose of antibiotics, was then hooked up while I waited for the scan. By now it was about 2:00 in the morning and so I called the substitute line to make sure that I had a sub to cover my class at school the next day.

School subs make up a very interesting group to study in human behavior. I can say this as I not only have worked with subs and my students tell me about them, but I also had subs way back when I was in school and I even was one for a time while waiting for a teaching opening and while working another job. First of all, in their defense, a sub gets absolutely no respect. When I was in school, we always gave the sub a hard time. Some things never change. And frankly, many subs gave off very strong reasons that justified making fun of them. Some looked kind of odd. Others smelled funny or had real bad breath. Others were retired teachers and they were quite mean. They were the ones who were grumpy, and they hated kids when they taught, and now that they were retired, they were even more grumpy. I never have understood why some people enter the teaching profession when they hate kids! These people give us a bad reputation! Then there were the subs that dressed a bit odd—like they just got off the boat at immigration central. Most subs would just pass on to the class the instructions that the teacher left for the day and then did their best to keep the students on task with gentle persuasion or through humorous reminders. These are the ones I like the best. Then there are the ones who became subs because they now have a captive audience to share their little political anecdotes or little philosophical gems that they have learned through their odd life experiences, or their little jokes that very rarely make sense, or others who like to give their two cents on their social views on topics ranging from politics to economics to others that are a bit more controversial—especially in a school setting—as in racist viewpoints or sexual innuendo or legalizing marijuana, sharing little gems of religion or anti-religion philosophies, and son on, and so on and so forth. These are the ones that I just wish would just pass on the instructions of the absent teacher and then just shut up and read the paper, or check out recent visitors to their UFO/Alien Encounter Face Book page, or the latest web site update on the buy-a-bride from Asia or Eastern Europe on the internet, or rolling a fatty underneath the teacher's desk, or whatever else they spend their time doing!

Our school used to have a sub that had to have been diagnosed with a very strong case of OCD (Obsessive-Compulsive Disorder). He would write these lengthy letters implicating students for sharing drinks, sharing Chapstick, sharing lotion, sharing food, sharing cell phones, or any other type of activity that would result in one student's stuff coming in any type of physical contact with another student—especially if it were to come in contact with any area of the face or mouth. He would write three to four pages per day of statements like, "I told Susan to stop sharing her bottled water with Jennifer. I warned them that they could get germs from each other and that it was not sanitary!!! Yet they did not heed my continued warnings and so I took their water away and called the security guard to come to the class and confiscate the water bottle." Or, "Johnny took off his shoe in class. I warned him that this was not sanitary, and to put his shoe back on, but he refused! So, I called security to come in and make sure that he put his shoe back on. After the security guard left, Johnny faked like he was going to take off his shoe again." He untied it, but he did not take it off. Of course, I warned him not to do so again as it violated the rules of sanitation of a safe and secure environment at school. He respected my wishes and did not attempt to take his shoe off again for the rest of the class." His lists went on and on with absurd stuff just like this so that by the end of the day, he had called security so many times, the school finally black listed him from ever coming back to the school. I used to love it when he covered my class because when I returned, I would always read his notes to the class. Sometimes I would even print them up and share them in an all-staff e-mail, so that the other staff members could share in the fun. These e-mails started quite a craze! They almost became a sort of news column that the staff could hardly wait to read the next episode. We all were a bit sad yet relieved when he got the boot.

Getting back to the story, I got an MRI and it showed lots of fluid in the surrounding tissue, but no evidence of infection or what the doctor referred to as puss pockets that they could treat or remove. And so soon after the antibiotic IV was drained, I was released to go back home.

Several weeks went by and the symptoms remained. They were beginning to get to me as I wasn't sleeping well, I was in a lot of pain and discomfort, and the doctors were puzzled as to what was the cause of my persisting condition. And, my surgeon's nurse was getting concerned that I was now hooked on the pain medication that I was continuing to take. And, since I was in pain, I was continuing to bother her for refills. Now I realize that I was getting hooked, but when you are in pain and there is no relief and you have a busy schedule to maintain, you not only begin to get a bit discouraged, but you start to get irritated that the medical profession begins to treat you as if you are a drug addict just persistently begging for your next fi x when in reality, you just want some relief to chronic pain that is making your life miserable as you try to stay focused at work while performing other duties at home as a husband and father. I knew full well that I would have to get off the pain meds through some kind of controlled treatment, but at that point I didn't give a crap about that. All I wanted was to get better and the pain to go away so that I could sleep and function somewhat more normally! My personal experience is that the medical field needs to distinguish between the abusers of the system and the patients in real need and then show an increased amount of compassion for those who really need the care. (Please wait just a minute as I get off my soap box!)

At about this time, I began to notice a little hair or stiff thread sticking out of my suture area. It was above the surface of the skin and it really bugged me. I asked my wife to look at it and she saw it also. She tried to pull it out with some tweezers, but she was pulling pretty hard and I didn't want her to tear any internal tissue, so I asked her to stop and I called the surgeon and asked them what I should do. They told me to come by and so I did and they cut it at the surface line of the skin and said that the rest should dissolve. They said that sometimes dissolving stitches don't always dissolve, and so the body will start to reject it and push it out—much like it would with an infected sliver that gets embedded underneath the skin, which the body naturally rejects and expels by itself. That made sense to me, so I went home hopeful that the rest of the stitch would work itself out and the infection would go away—thus alleviating my problems. Unfortunately for me, it wasn't that simple. And so, after several more weeks of the stitch continuing to poke out, I decided to go to the hospital and have the rest of it taken out by a doctor—even if it was still inside the skin. And frankly, I didn't care how deep it was. I was tired of dealing with it. So, this next time I decided to go to the hospital, before I went, I called my friend who works there in the ER and made sure that he was on duty. His wife told me that he was at the hospital and so I drove down to the hospital to have him take a look and do some probing and poking around. The nice thing about having my friend there was that I would make sure and say "Hi" when I arrived, and he would always ignore the patients who had checked in before me and call me in ahead of the rest. It's kind of cool to get the VIP treatment at the ER room. I guess that it's kind of like getting seconds for dinner in prison. He took a look at it and he asked me if I would mind if he cut the skin and see how deep the stitch went and to remove it. I told him to go ahead and cut the dang thing out—regardless of how deep it was. But I recommended that he stop cutting if he got all the way to my penis. He assured me he would stop at that point and I assured him that I was joking—unless the thing did go all the way to my thing at which point I would ask that he stop doing the thing he was doing! We had a nice laugh as he started to cut. He ended up removing about an eighth of an inch of stitch. He said that the tissue around the stitch looked good and that he couldn't see any puss or infection. He asked me if I was okay with him doing some probing in the surrounding tissue with a syringe to see if he could locate any other infection. I told him to go ahead and he did so with no luck. There was no apparent infection. As he stitched me up, he told me that I should se an infectious disease specialist to get this what appeared to be infection treated. So, I thanked him and went home to await the red tape from a request to my primary care provider to refer me to an ID specialist.

In the meantime, my surgeon felt it time for me to get off my pain meds and so he gave me a referral to another pain management specialist. I wanted to see the first one I went to after the fusion, but my primary care provide wouldn't approve him. After all, he actually did know what he was doing, and he treated me with dignity and respect, but he was no longer included in my medical group, and so I was sent to another office, and of course, I did not see the actual doctor for whom the office is named. Rather, I saw one of his PA's. And if I didn't know better, I would have thought that she was hired right out of her previous position of teaching preschoolers. But, she was nice and very, very considerate. She was big on building my self-esteem and using a very uplifting positive vocabulary—a technique she practiced with her previous toddlers and perfected through a medical training seminar entitled something like "Building a Trusting Relationship With Your Drug Addict Patients Through the Use of Nurturing Words of Tender Positive Reassurance Reinforced With the Special Technique of Utilizing Kind and Reassuring Facial Expressions, Appropriate Shoulder Taps, and Non-Offensive Body Gestures." About halfway through the visit, I thought she was going to dim the lights, pull out her visual aids of pop-up medical books, and read me a story while I sat on a little rug eating graham crackers and drinking orange juice. But since I was tired of the side effects of the meds and I was willing and had a desire to stop, I met with her on two separate occasions while I stepped down and off the meds in about a month. I am not so sure that her seminar training had a lot to do with my stopping—although I bet she felt so proud of herself that she took the seminar instead of going out to party with the rest of her office group while at the medical conference. Actually, the key to the success was my willingness and desire to stop. That is the key to success in situations such as these.

Now, I was off the pain medication, but the symptoms continued. My referral finally came through for me to see the infectious disease specialist. Once again, I felt encouraged that a cure was close at hand. That is like T-Rex thinking that the little snow storm would soon pass and that the weather was about to change—right at the onset of the ice age!

So, the referral came and I was requested to get some preliminary lab work done prior to the appointment. At this point I had been dealing with this so-called infection for about six months. Fortunately, this time I actually saw the doctor whose name was on the front door. And, I was very lucky too since he only had office hours three hours a week! And so, even though his nurse triple books patients and fortunately for me they were stocked with year old People Magazines, Golf Digests (I am not a golfer), Highlights magazines (I remember reading about Tommy Timbertoes when I was a kid and I did like to find the hidden pictures within the picture in Highlight, but that was when I was about five. The waiting room was also filled with other miscellaneous magazines specifically subscribed to by doctors as a way of furthering torture on defenseless patients. Once I met with this doctor, he felt confident that I did have an infection of some kind and he ordered some more blood work, a bone scan called a Gallium Scan, and he ordered me an aggressive plan of IV antibiotics for two or three months. This required getting a pick line placed in my arm by the hospital's nuclear medicine department (kind of like the x-ray guys), so that I could give myself an IV bag of antibiotics at home twice a day for two months to finally kill the beast! (This made me twinge just a bit as you may remember my experience with the last pick line I had right after my gall bladder surgery!) So, for the next two and a half months, I received a delivery of medical supplies at my home so that I could give myself the IV's every morning for an hour before work, and every night about 12 hours later before I went to bed. Then, I had a home care nurse come once a week to check my vitals, draw some blood, and clean the dressing around the pick line. This wasn't so bad except that I had to get up an hour early every morning to do the IV drip. And the antibiotics made me nauseous and tired. And, they were full of sodium, which did not help my diet plan much. But, I got used to the routine and I would do anything at this point to rid myself of this very stubborn phantom infection. During the IV period, the infectious disease doctor wanted me to get a test done to see if he could locate the source of the infection, and so he requested a Gallium Scan. This test was done by injecting me with a radio-active dye that over time, would cluster around areas of bacteria. I was injected with the dye and then over the next three days, a scan was done with an imaging machine similar to an MRI that would locate the areas of concentrated dye in order to find out the exact location of the so-called infection. The test was completed, and the results forwarded to the infectious disease doctor. He called me in for a follow up visit and told me that there was no evidence that I had a bacterial infection. Next, he cancelled my IV's and submitted an order to my home care provider to remove the pick line. Then, he recommended that I go back to my neurosurgeon for further consultation, and he told me that he would be glad to provide me with a referral for a second opinion, provided I could figure out who I was supposed to be referred to. Finally, he then wished me luck and sent me on my way to find help somewhere else. I was beginning to feel like I was running out of options, and that perhaps I should be searching the Yellow Pages for a witch doctor or voodoo practitioner.

I returned to my surgeon who took another look at the red, swollen area on my back and he felt confident that this was a viral infection of the nerve close to the incision area. He put me on some very strong antiviral medication for the next two weeks. I took five big horse pills a day for ten days. You may be able to guess the results of this new idea—right you are! Nada, Zip, Zilch!

Ten months had now passed by and I was still at ground zero. But, the symptoms were beginning to flare up so that at night my back would get hot and I would get hot. While I needed the windows open and all the fans blowing on high speed, my wife was walking around the house with sweatshirts and blankets on. And, I was well into my daily routine of coming home from work, placing my feather pillow on my recliner in front of the TV, and while placing an ice pack (I had three) on my pillow, I would sit back and ice my back while watching TV. Thank goodness for DVR! And if you asked my wife, she would say that I lived in that chair! And she was pretty much right on! I lived at work and then came home to the chair.

Through all this, I had picked up a great trick to try to cool myself off at night. Have you ever heard of the term of being cool like the other side of the pillow? Do you ever rotate your pillow at night to feel the cool side of the pillow? Well I do. My problem is that the other side absolutely cannot cool off fast enough! So, I figured out that when I went to bed, I could place an ice pack in between my two pillows. Then, as the pillow warmed up, I would switch sides and the other side would be ice-cold from the ice pack! Ingenious—right! I know for a fact that there is someone out there reading this and shouting with sheer and utter joy as this little revelation has lifted the clouds of ignorance in dealing with hot-head sleeping disorder! Don't worry—no need to thank me. You bought this book! Just go out and buy the large gel-filled ice bag, freeze it, and enjoy a wonderful night's sleep!

I returned once again to my surgeon after he had requested, and I had gone in to get another MRI. He looked it over and over. He examined my back very carefully. He re-questioned me as to all of the symptoms that I was feeling, and then he came to the conclusion that my spine was fi ne. He continued to tell me that he thought that what I was suffering from was an autonomic vascular disorder of some kind, and he told me that he was going to refer me to one of two specialists in this area. So once again I left his office and once again I placed my life in the hands of my primary care provider while I waited for the approval process to take its course. The irony here is that during this very exact week, my work's annual medical insurance renewal was taking place and I had the opportunity, if I so chose, to change medical plans. And, it may shock you when I tell you that my wife and I were actually thinking about changing plans. However, if we were to do so, I would have to start completely over and go see another set of doctors for this condition. And, since I had already invested ten months in this very volatile relationship, I was not about to start over from scratch. I have heard that in typical relationships, the standard advice is to be that just because you are in a relationship a long time, there is absolutely no sense in sticking it out simply because you have invested a lot of time, energy, emotion and money. The advice would be to get out immediately! Well perhaps I was in too deep to see clearly, but I decided to stick with my good old primary care provider partner, even though I had some pretty strong suspicions that she was cheating on me the whole time—just for my money!

So, as of the writing of these memoirs, I still have not found a solution to my problem. I am hoping that the next doctor or specialist I see will hold the knowledge of the secret to my healing so that I can finally feel better and be healed, whatever that means. But what if that doesn't happen? What if I will have chronic pain issues the rest of my life—what then? Well, the last chapter discusses my plan along with some advice for others who have health challenges like I have had. But I will say this—I am not going to go out and order a roll-away bed and check myself into a long-term, self-diagnosed home health care plan, quit work, say my final good-byes to family and friends, and start to die! I have a lot of good years ahead—and I mean a lot of wonderful memories yet to create, and I am not about to give in and give up when it comes to dealing with poor health issues. Instead, I am going to "pucker up my sphincter" as my old high school football coach used to say, and get on with life with a smile on my face, humor in my heart, and a joke on my lips!

Chapter 8

Aging and Urination. A Delicate Topic for Delicate Times

I would like to talk to you today about aging and urination. From a male's perspective, the practice of urination remains fairly normal through the age of 45. At about 40, there are some warning signs that you may be experiencing what I call, F U, or frequent urination. For example, if you are watching s super hero movie and you need to go number one right at the climax of the movie. Or, you are in a traffic jam on the freeway and have to pee so bad that you drive on the shoulder amidst horn honking and middle finger pointing all the way to the next exit, where you speed up the off-ramp and pull into the first rat hole service station you come to, then jump out and use sign language with the non-English speaking attendant and demand to use the bathroom. The attendant gives you a key attached to a two-foot long galvanized pipe and desperately trying to open the old door, that has had numerous break in attempts by homeless people looking for a restroom, your trembling hands finally open the door to a filthy room full of stench. Taking a deep breath, and not caring that there is a pile of paper towels and fecal matter piled up in the toilet, you run in and use the urinal—which does not look much better. You finish, attempt a flush that has long since had running water, then run outside and exhale then gasp for breath.

If this is your situation, then you have the preliminary stages of F U!

When a man turns 45, he gets his first prostate check. A prostate check is something that makes most males uncomfortable to say the least. The prostate is a vital part of a male's hydraulic system. It allows the elevator to get all the way up to the top floor—if you know what I mean. For me, when I turned 45, my insurance had two urologists to choose from. I had heard that both were good, so what I did was I went to their office and met each one in person, shaking hands with each one and in doing so, taking a mental note of each of their hand sizes. After that, the choice was easy.

One of the doctors had big calloused hands with large, thick fingers. His voice was loud and intimidating. He also had sort of a strange grin—a grin that made me feel a bit uncomfortable. The other doctor had small, more delicate hands with shorter, narrow fingers. He was also soft-spoken and kind—very polite. After meeting both, my choice was obvious. I chose the second doctor. I waited in the waiting room for my visit, all the while having this feeling that I had a wedgie. However, when I reached to fix the wedgie, it wasn't there. I had experienced a P W, or in other words, a phantom wedgie! I made the assumption that while waiting to get his prostate checked, a male could experience a P W.

The nurse showed me to the exam room, where I was to await the doctor. As I sat there, I began to read all the medical posters.
These were quite educational and yet somewhat disturbing.

While I read, I found myself squirming in my seat. It seems that my sphincter was getting anxious. I guess he sort of felt like a prize fighter who had already been introduced in the ring and was waiting for the round one bell to ring. One poster had a diagram of an enlarged prostate. Another showed details of an inflamed hemorrhoid, while a third displayed detail of erectile dysfunction.

After squirming through a couple of rounds of viewing posters, the doctor entered the office. We shook hands again and again, I was grateful that his hand in mine was not much larger than a child's hands. Yet being a father, I knew that a child's small hands could still get into a lot of trouble and wreak much havoc!

The doctor politely asked me to pull down my trousers—I liked the fact that he used the word trousers—it seemed to reduce the tension in the room—just a bit. While the doctor put on the blue gloves, he asked me to drop my shorts and lean over the examination table. Now I am not quite sure why the gloves are blue. Perhaps it is because the patient—me—was holding his breath so long in anticipation of the insertion that the skin on his face turned a pale shade of blue. As I turned my head to take a breath, I saw that the doctor had placed a generous amount of lubricating gel on his fingers. As he rubbed the gel into the gloves with his fingers, I began to hyper-ventilate.

At this point of the exam, I decided it best to turn around and look straight ahead, preferring a surprise to knowing the exact time of finger insertion. Perhaps I was thinking that this was sort of like getting in a car wreck. If the victim knows he is going to get hit, he tenses up so much, that on impact, his muscles are much more damaged than if he did not see the wreck coming and thus, being more relaxed, would experience less injury. Besides in this case, if my rectal muscles were to be flexed and rigid, it would have made his finger entry sort of like hitting one of those concrete road construction barriers, resulting in a total shut down of the on-ramp. Fortunately, it didn't take long for the episode to occur. I am a bit foggy on the details, but I do remember having sort of an out of body experience where I was visiting a maximum-security prison full of hard core criminals—very lonely criminals!

I reentered my body and pulled up my shorts. I looked at the doctor, experiencing some feelings that reminded me of my first date in high school. Sheepishly, I told the doctor that now we had made a special connection, I felt compelled to ask him out for dinner. He politely turned me down. I found myself feeling a little bit disappointed, although not sure why. I shook his hand—now glove free—and told him that I looked forward to seeing him in a year. I enjoyed our annual rendezvous for five years until I hit the wall of turning fifty.

Inevitably, unless you have Superman powers to reverse the rotation of the earth and go back in time, you now reach the milestone of half a century. You turn fifty years old. You have now passed the point of no return. You have a foggy recollection of your past, and you are beginning to resist your future, knowing that you have now lived longer than the life you have left. At fifty, when you are watching the super hero movie, and you have a soda and popcorn, and you do make it to the climax of the movie, you suddenly have the overwhelming urge to go to the bathroom so bad that you can feel your rapidly escalating pulse in your private! When your pulse hits about 120 BPM's, you realize that you have about thirty seconds to get to the potty. Then, as you go and go and go, and the stream that is normally little more than a trickle is now flowing like a racehorse and with such velocity that the splash is peppering your clothes like you just visited Niagara Falls, as you finish and do that little ritual to rid your private of any residual liquid, you feel a shudder of such intense pleasure, that your knees buckle and you have to grab the wall to prevent yourself from collapsing, you realize that you haven't felt this ecstatic rush for years!

At fifty, you find that you can no longer buy a Super Big Gulp—even on a hot day and especially when you are driving on busy freeways such as those found in Southern California. For if you do buy the big drink, and you do get stuck in traffic, and there is no exit in sight, you find yourself rolling down the window, pouring out the remainder of the soda onto the pavement, and then doing something so desperate, that you cannot tell a soul what you have done—even your poker buddies after sharing a 24-pak. First, you situate your car so that the cars on either side of you are not lined up directly to your side. And of course, you make sure that there are no trucks and especially no semi-trucks at your side. (Truck drivers sit real high in their seat with a good view of drivers in their cars below.) Then you remove the lid of your large cup and you arch your back, making your back rigid and level with your legs. Then you unzip and drain your maximum- capacity bladder into the cup. Yes, you are so desperate that you do the unthinkable. You pee in the soda cup!

Unfortunately, you must repeat the process at least two more times before you get out of the heavy traffic. For some reason, when you open those flood gates, they simply do not nor cannot nor will not shut off. And once you are finished, and your back is still rigid because you are trying your best to empty the hose— sort of like when you are topping off your gas tank and you know that there is still a little more gas in the hose so you keep tapping the nozzle against your gas orifice, and even after tapping and tapping, when you go to put the hose away a trickle of gas spurts out—the same thing happens when you relax your back and sit back down. For now, your nozzle is now lower than your bladder and gravity sets in, leaving a nice puddle on your pants—sure to be noticed at your destination—even if it is quite a distance away. For those of you who wish to pass judgment on this action, and you think that perhaps this is gross or disgusting or below the dignity of a human being, know this—Unless you have been so helplessly desperate that you would literally sell your soul to the devil for a toilet, or if you had to pee so bad that your private parts felt like an over-inflated water balloon about to explode, and leaving your private part blown apart like a cartoon cigar, then please show just a little bit of compassion.

At age fifty, your basketball game that you once had in high school—not your shot, for your shot goes even wilder, but your dribble returns with a passion. And, no matter how you wrap up your peeing experience, whether you shake or tap or thump or slap or tickle or wiggle or twist or wring out, or even if you scream at it as if scaring it would make it stop like the hiccups, there is still a dribble or trickle or drip down the front of your pants. Now, when you use a public restroom, and typically you look for paper towels as you absolutely loathe those damn air dryers, you seek out these inventions of Satan, for now you use these dryers to try and dry off the wet stain that has run down the front of your pants!

Also at fifty years old, with no other alternative, and with some kind of sick desire to return to the very man who traumatized you five years ago by violating your rectal area, you go back to Doctor Small Hands and ask for a prescription for some pills that somehow either enlarge your bladder, or magically increase your control, or perhaps as a placebo, strengthen your resolve for more control.

The next milestone, or should I say gallstone as it was at this age when my gallbladder died inside of me and began to spread gangrene throughout my vital organs that almost killed me and caused me severe discomfort and a prolonged stay in the hospital losing 28 pounds in nine days, is turning fifty-five. At fifty-five, you now get up three to four times a night to pee. And, while you are up, you may find yourself semi-consciously heading to the kitchen where you make a quick search for any stray snacks that are within reach and require little effort to snatch up and take back to bed with you. The problem with that is that there may be times when you take a cookie or a piece of chocolate candy or even an ice cream bar back to bed with you, and before you eat it all, you fall back asleep. When that happens, especially with anything that can melt with body heat, you wake up the next morning laying in a puddle of melted mess! When this occurs, you have no alternative but to let your spouse know that someone must have entered your house during the night, gone to the kitchen for a snack, then came in to your bedroom and while looming over you and eating your food, they considered slitting your throat and robbing you of all your valuables. At that point, when your spouse begins to laugh uncontrollably and call you on your B.S. story, then you must face the music and confess that you had a little accident or mishap in your sleep, but you only confess that you had been sleep walking or sleep walk-snacking at the time of the incident for which you have n recollection. This story will make its way through all of the family get-togethers, Thanksgiving dinners, and summer vacations. Your children and other relatives will laugh at you and ridicule you while you nod your head and grin, appearing to go along with their mockery. I guess it's not so bad. After all, it is great to get together with your kids—even if your story is the biggest hit of the event.

At fifty-five, your two little buddies down there that used to serve a vital purpose in the propagation of your family name, now pass on to permanent retirement. These two guys, who once were packed snugly into their little mummy bag, now swing freely on their hammock, without a care in the world. For this reason, a man must now graduate from wearing regular gym shorts, to extra-long Jordan shorts. If a fifty-five-year-old male were to wear shorts with a regular rise in the inseam, then those around him may have an unexpected surprise in the works when this individual sits down and opens his knees. I shudder at the very thought!

Another way to describe this situation is through an analogy. Those of you who are a bit older may remember a novelty toy called "Clackers." Clackers were two glass-like balls that had a 12inch string running through each of the balls that came together and led to a small round plastic circle that you could hold onto. Then, if you moved your hand up and down, the two balls on the string would go up and down, making a "clack" sound as they hit. When a person got good at this, they could clack the clackers back and forth for an extended period of time, and in doing so, be the life of the party. Of course, if the clackers were the only party games that you provided for your big party, people would come to the party, eat the food, see the clacker game, then quickly make up an excuse that the babysitter just called, and the kids got sick on some bad pizza and they take off.

If you don't get the innuendo, I will give it one more shot with another analogy. If you are too young to remember Clackers, then perhaps you are familiar with the Sharper Image catalog, or perhaps stores that sell executive type gifts for the guy who has everything. If you are familiar with this type of product, then you may know about those gifts with the stacks of steelies, or silver balls that hang from strings on a wooden frame. When you swing one, it comes back and hits the stack of steelies, causing the steelie on the opposite end to pop out. Then, the steelies clack back and forth until the resistance brings them to a stop. If you still don't know what I am talking about, then I am going to have to hit you right between the eyes with a very direct and obvious explanation. But once I do this, don't come back and say that this is gross, or something like that. So, here goes...get ready...Okay. If when you sit down for a number two, and you can not only FEEL water, but you can also tell that there is some depth to the water, then you now understand what I am talking about. This is fifty-five.

You may be asking yourself, "Why is he mentioning this? What does it have to do with urination?" Well, since you brought it up, I will tell you why.

I have a close relative, and just as the television crime documentaries change the names of the victims to protect the innocent, I will give this relative the name "Fred." According to multiple sources and again, when doing a documentary, the name "Fred." According to multiple sources, Fred's wife insists, no demands that Fred sit down when he goes number one. Again, when doing a documentary, it is important for accuracy sake to have multiple sources —especially of you have no eye witnesses. If this is true about Fred, and I believe that it is, I must call upon men everywhere to unite! Men, regardless of any political, philosophical or religious differences that we may have, we must unite as one voice and "take a stand!"

We must draw a line in the sand and even at the risk of losing our very manhood—that instinctive force that has been genetically passed down from generations past all the way back to our cave man progenitors who clubbed their women then dragged them back inside the cave—declare that we will not, we cannot yea, we shall not, under any circumstance and even at the risk of sacrificing all that we have including our very lives, ever, NEVER sit down to pee! For if we do my brothers, we are nothing more than sheep on their way to the slaughterhouse, lemmings on their way to a cliff, male-gendered pieces of meaningless flesh, with nothing left to identify our manhood. To give in to such a demand would signify that our very testicles have been removed and we are nothing more than Eunuchs, something slightly less than human, an animated manikin if you will, to be used and abused, until there is no further purpose that justifies it's pathetic existence, to then be discarded by the wayside—thrown off to the side of the highway—weighed down by rocks and sunk into the sea - by the female gender.

If we are given the request of squatting on the throne, then we take a stand and deal with the consequences accordingly! This defining moment of manhood is a black or white issue. There is no grey area—no room for interpretation—no excuse or exception—not today, not ever.

With that oath firmly resolved in our souls, I shall move on to discuss night urination. Unfortunately, the aging male population does not have access to infrared or night vision goggles for urination. I think that Wal-Mart could have a great product on their hands if they could offer this kind of product for sale for men to use as they urinate at night. However, they would need to drop the price and they would have to design the product so that it could somehow be placed or strapped on the head quickly and easily, and it would probably need to come with an accessory like a wall-hanging hook so that a guy could hang it right by the bed for quick accessibility. Sadly, there is no such thing as this nocturnal male urinary device so we must move on.

When you, as an aging gentleman, wake up in the middle of the night to go potty or go and do a fly by in the kitchen for a quick snack, and because you are now getting out of bed so frequently, you learn to make it to the bathroom without turning on the light. Your intentions are good. You don't want to wake up your spouse—even though she is snoring up a storm—but sometimes you end up walking into the wall or stubbing your toe on the wall in which case, you may just slip out a few expletives, which may wake up the spouse anyway, depending on which words escape your mouth.

Anyway, let's say that you make it to the bathroom and step inside. Now, you line up for your blind shot at hitting the water— or at least hit the inside of the porcelain. Unfortunately, sometimes even the best of intentions go terribly wrong. Therefore, in order to do my part to pass on some advice to those of you who may end up, sooner or later, attempting to pee in the middle of the night without turning on the light, I have been able to identify and describe the different sounds that could be created when a stream of urine strikes different types of surfaces in the toilet area. So, here are the descriptions that match up the surface with the sound of urine striking that surface.

There you are, in the dark, standing in front of the toilet. You have touched the sides of your mid-calf against the bowl in order to get your bearings and line yourself up in front of the toilet. Maybe of you are like me, you have placed your hand on the wall at your side to double check your position. I have done this so frequently that over time, I have completely rubbed the paint off the wall in the shape of a handprint. Now it is time to give a little abdominal push and initiate urine flow. Remember that once this happens, there is no turning back. The next moment is critical in determining whether or not you have struck your target, or you will be forced to turn on the light in order to see for your necessary clean-up on the collateral damage area—however extensive and wherever that may be.

Next, you release the fluid and you listen to see which surface your urine is striking. If at this point you hear nothing, you are probably in serious trouble and it means one of two things. First, it is conceivable that you are shooting blanks—no fluid is being discharged. Although highly unlikely, this has been known to happen—especially when it is the middle of the night and you are considerably drowsy. You may possibly be in a lucid dream state where you are dreaming that you are urinating when in reality, you are not. When you realize that this is happening, shake your head back into conscious awareness and give a good abdominal push and flow will commence.

The other alternative if you hear nothing is not good. If you know that fluid is flowing, then this means that your stream is hitting the floor—if you have vinyl flooring in the bathroom. If you have tile flooring, you may hear a sound I can best describe as a sort of dribble-splat-splatter sound. If you hear this sound or if you hear nothing, commence emergency shutdown procedures and do everything in your power to bring all flow to an abrupt halt. Urinating on the floor—even for a very short period of time—results in a considerable amount of clean up area when you are through. For some reason, when urine hits the floor, it begins to spread out quickly and containment is very difficult. I recommend—and this may be easier said than done—that you shut down the procedure, roll out as much toilet paper you can as fast as you can, and begin wiping down the floor immediately, before the puddle becomes a pond or worse—a lake! Do a quick containment wipe-down, then finish your business. Before returning to bed, make sure that the door is closed and turn on the light so that you can see good enough to wipe up the rest of the liquid.

If you do not shut the door, your wife may wake up when you turn on the light. If so, then she will surely ask you what happened in the bathroom and you will have to give her one of two explanations. The first is telling the truth, which she does not like to hear because by now she is very tired of doing the bathroom clean-up with the Comet and the other cleaning products necessary to get the job done correctly. The other alternative is that you will have to make something up to explain why you had to turn on the light. I can give you a few excuses I have used in the past, but even after your best attempt to cover up the truth, inevitably her response will still be to ask you, in a condescending and accusatory tone, if you have peed on the floor again. Anyway, here are a few excuses you can try, but remember, you have to do your best to sound convincing, which can be challenging in the middle of the night:

1. We were out of toilet paper and I had to change the roll.
2. Oh honey, you would not believe it but I had another episode of acid reflux and I had to get up and take a pill!

3. It's awful, dear; I think that the chicken I ate was bad. I thought I had to throw up!

4. Here is some tissue honey. (Sound sympathetic and loving and hand her some toilet paper which means that some advance planning is necessary.) You were sniffling in your sleep and it sounded like you may be getting a cold! Then throw in a little sweet comment like "Honey, do you know how much I love you and care about you?" Then, give her a kiss on the cheek and cuddle with her a while. After rubbing her back gently several times, then you can carefully return to your sleeping position on your side of the bed—just don't be in a rush during this critical procedure as she may think you to be insensitive, in which case this whole elaborate scheme is all for naught. This technique can only be used once a year and during cold season.

One little tip here: whichever excuse you try, keep it brief. The more you talk, the more your wife will wake up and the more she wakes up, the better her thinking processes will become and the greater the likelihood that she will realize that you are covering up the fact that you have once again urinated on HER floor.

Now let's get back to identifying the different noises.

If you hear a low-pitched thudding noise, then unfortunately my friend, your aim is way off. You have struck the rubber on the toilet plunger located off to the side in the back corner. If that happens, you have one or two alternatives. You can either shut off the flow, which in the middle of the night can be very difficult, and then re-adjust and try again, or you simply rotate your hips in the direction of the toilet and listen for the desired splashing sound. At this point do not, and I repeat DO NOT readjust by moving your feet. If you do so, the errant spray will shoot up and down looking something like the lines of an EKG. Thus, your clean-up will include everything from floor to underside of lid and that little space in between the bowl and the tank.

The next sound you may hear is a loud thumping ricochet-like sound. If you hear this, your urine has struck the plastic container that holds the toilet brush. If this happens, refer to the instructions above and follow the same procedure as if you had struck the plunger. The next sound you may hear once your flow has commenced is a mid-range pitched hollow echo. If you hear this, your aim is too high. Your flow is hitting the underside of the toilet lid. Because it takes so much self-control and can cause a considerable amount of pain in shutting down the flow at this point, and the results will still involve clean up in the exact same area because as you shut off the flow it is sort of like turning off a garden hose with the flow slowly reducing until it is completely shut off, it is best at this point to either bend at the hips and lean forward or redirect the "hose" if you will, and continue the drainage without interruption.

The next possible sound you could hear, and frankly this would be a more welcome sound is a quieter glassy-hissing sound. If you hear this sound, you have struck the porcelain of the bowl which means one of two things. Either you are striking the rim of the bowl or you have at last hit the inside of the bowl. If the latter happens, you are okay. You may want to make controlled minute adjustments to see of you can't hear the splashing of water inside the bowl. If the former, you are in somewhat of a volatile predicament. If you adjust the stream in the wrong direction, and you hear nothing, then you are now peeing on the floor. As stated above, this is bad and requires considerable clean-up. If however, you adjust in the right direction, you will recognize the sound of striking the inside of the bowl or a splashing sound—both mean that you have found your way to the target. Once there, continue your business until you have finished. I must interject one last point here. As your flow diminishes, for some reason and even if you are standing directly at the front of the bowl, and it appears that even if the urine at this angle was directed straight down you could not miss the bowl, you will end up dribbling on the floor. To avoid this, simply rotate your hips forward and slightly adjust your stance so that you are leaning slightly more over the bowl. At this point, I always listen for the pitter-patter of drops hitting the floor, and even if I hear no sound, I still check the floor to see if there are any drops of splatter. If I find any, and I almost always do, I wipe them up before they dry. Otherwise, an accumulation of these dried drops will cause a negative reaction by your spouse. (Perhaps I should use the word "strained," or "distressful," or maybe even the words "agonizingly painful," instead of the word "negative" in that previous sentence.)

If a clean-up procedure is necessary, then here are a few tips: First, you have to shut the door, turn on the light and assess the crime scene. You might think that the word "crime" is stretching it a bit, but I assure you that when a man pees anywhere but inside the toilet, but even then, there is collateral damage from splashing, then his wife considers this a criminal act! So, take a little time and look at the critical areas—the areas that tick your wife off the most because they are the most difficult to clean. Here is a list of these critical areas:

1. The small space in between the tank and the bowl. If this area has been contaminated, then take about a foot of toilet paper, fold it in half or thirds, depending on how wide the gap is, and slide the paper inside the gap, allowing enough time to absorb the fluid inside this area.

2. The underside of the lid and bowl. If so, simply wipe down all drippage.

3. The small crack in the floor between the tile and the bowl. This is a critical area to clean for if it is neglected, over time, it will become discolored and even (if you have some kind of vinyl flooring) cause the tile to lift off the concrete surface underneath. This is not good, and you will be blamed for it!

4. Collateral damage: The floor all around the base of the bowl including and especially behind the bowl. If your hit and miss tactics resulted in urinating on the floor, and you know that the puddle had enough time to turn into a pond or a lake, then there is sure to be some fluid on the floor behind the bowl. If this is not cleaned and is allowed to dry, it will leave a discolored residue that requires cleanser to be removed. The wife does not appreciate this! When she is forced to bring out the cleanser and scrub, all of her past emotions and frustrations of past episodes having to clean up after you come to her conscious thoughts and as she cleans, they build an emotional momentum in her head, crescendoing with her gritting of teeth and mumbling to herself,

sounding like a hissing snake that is ready to strike. When this happens, it is like an emotional steam valve bursting with a blast of hot billowing vaporous slander that once released, can include years and even decades worth of pent in complaints. If by chance you walk by and hear this happening, let it go—let her vent. This is a healthy release. Just as the release of a steam valve prevents an explosion of pressurized steam, her emotional release at this time prevents her from exploding at you—a spewing of past complaints, regrets and disappointments which you do not want to hear. So, if you hear this in progress, get out! Run! But do not let her hear you in the area. If she does, she will call you out (or should I say "in") and demand that you come in and watch her clean up the mess and see what she has to go through every time you pee on the floor. Listening to this raving may go on for an extended period of time so be patient and understanding. Take it like a man.

If by chance, at this point, she begins to cry, drop to your knees immediately! Put your arm around her, tell her that you are deeply sorry, insist that you finish the clean up and tell her how much you love and appreciate her. If you do so sincerely, in her vulnerability she will smile with a renewed appreciation for your sensitivity and tell you that she will finish but she appreciates your thoughtfulness. If this happens, kiss her, tell her again how much she means to you, then get out of there quickly, for just as your Pit Bull can be your best friend one moment and attack you with deadly force in the next, this moment of fragile vulnerability will not last long. So get out of the area, go to the family room, turn on the TV and stay out of her way. When she is finished, tell her that you have reservations for dinner at her favorite restaurant and take her out that very evening. After all, it could be a lot worse! And, you get a nice meal out of the deal!

I should interject one more important point if you have a tile flooring with grout in between the tiles. This grout also will discolor over time. I recommend that if you see this area is darker—meaning that it is wet and has been contaminated, you go and get the cleanser and make a greater effort to clean this area. Remember that "an ounce of prevention is worth a pound of cure."

I will and I must discuss one final point, and I will approach this subject most delicately. During this whole transition of nocturnal urination once a man hits that mystical age of forty, there may be times—although not nearly as frequently as in earlier years—when urinating at night in the dark, there may be what I would call "crime scene exit closure." If you are puzzled by this title, I will attempt to give further explanation, while maintaining a high degree of discretion. If you have seen a crime scene in person or on television, you know that in order to maintain the integrity of the scene, and for the sake of discussion let's say that a mass murder occurred inside a family residence, there would be a bright yellow or sometimes red tape stretched across the door at a variety of angles to block any outside force from entry into the house. Even the tape itself carries a message in bold capital letters that reads, "CRIME SCENE DO NOT ENTER."

There may be times when we just might have some fi gurative crime scene tape stretched across the "exit" of our urinary flow. And, just as a scene of a horrifi c, brutal crime, and let's say for the sake of the analogy that there was a shot gun involved, (I do not wish to get too graphic but I do need to give a clear image of what I am talking about.) then when the guns discharge, there will be splatter.

If this is the case, do not attempt to remove the crime scene tape while continuing to trespass the criss-crossing tape and break into the crime scene. If you do, there will be severe splatter. All you can do at this point is stop immediately and remove the tape. This will allow for un-obstructive exit. If you do not understand this analogy, I am sorry but it's the best I could come up with, so too bad.

P.S. If you find yourself in a Code Red situation where no matter how you adjust your feet and your hip rotation, and you have already heard each of the dribble-splat-splatter, low-pitched thudding, thumping ricochet and/or a mid-range pitched hollow echo sounds meaning that you have a considerable contamination area on the floor, and you have done your very best to clean up the mess including a follow up inspection and wipe down check the following morning, and the toilet area still smells like a truck stop bathroom outside of Winnemucca Nevada, then you need to check the horse-shoe shaped rug that surrounds the toilet. You know, the cute little rug that comes in a variety of fabrics, textures and color schemes all designed for the purpose of making that toilet area somehow magically appear to look "cute," or "pretty," or even "quaint." Now I personally believe that you cannot polish a turd. And even though the television program that proves clichés such as this to be inaccurate, I still believe that you cannot polish a turd. A toilet is still a toilet. And even if your toilet has been imported from Italy or is made from a special hand-blown porcelain made especially for you by a Tibetan monk, it is still just a device that is used to discharge number one or number two or sometimes both.

However, if after clean-up there is a strong, lingering scent of urine, then smell the rug. (Or to be more specific, the toilet floor mat.) If it smells like the ten-year-old once white, now brownish green mop that sits in the corner of that Winnemucca truck stop bathroom closet, then simply take to the laundry room when your wife isn't looking and stick it in the washing machine and after adding the proper amount of detergent, start it up. Then when your wife asks you if you are doing some laundry, simply tell her that you thought you'd help her out and put in a load of your dirty clothes so that more of her time can be freed up to garden or knit or write poetry. She will think that you are so sweet and considerate! Then, while she is perfecting her new hobby, slip the newly washed rug in the dryer before she does, to avoid her discovery of the contents inside the machine. When it is dry, and your wife is off doing errands or perhaps planting some tulips in the garden, then go get the cute little rug and replace it to its proper place surrounding the toilet. Now, the smell of urine should no longer be present. And you also have the fresh smell of your "Spring Fresh Scented" laundry detergent as an added deterrent of bad odors!

Men, I have discussed a topic that few dared to put on paper. Most of this subject matter has only been discussed in soft tones among camping buddies or bowling teams after a few brewskies. However, I felt it my duty, nay, my obligation as a fellow male passing through the advancing years of life, to put this information to paper. I do so at the expense of my own pride and self-dignity. This matters not to me if doing so may in some way provide a life-saving buoy ring to some poor soul who has fallen overboard in the treacherous seas of marital difficulties as a result of the high tides and treacherous currents of urinary dysfunction. All I ask is that if you are fortunate enough to receive this information, that you share it with another poor soul who unbeknownst to you, has fallen victim to this challenging and debilitating obstacle of aging.

To all the men everywhere who have ever had to get up to pee in the middle of the night, and who do so without the lights on, I salute you!

Chapter 9

So, My Health Is Shot. What Do I Do Now?

As I have traveled this rocky journey of health challenges, I feel that I have learned some very valuable lessons that have helped me deal with them and still remain active with the things that I really want to do. I have managed to keep a positive outlook on life and the activities that I am involved in including work and family. And I look forward to many more wonderful years of personal fulfillment and fun sharing in all of the wonderful adventures that lie ahead with work, friends, family and soon to be grandkids as my wife and I reach the early afternoon hours of our earthly existence. In doing so, I would like to share with you some advice that has helped me get through the some of the more difficult health challenges I have had with a smile on my face, and with a positive outlook in my head. I call this my natural prescription for life. This prescription is made up of six tips that if followed, will bring you greater personal happiness and well-being. In sharing these suggestions, I'm afraid that I will place my humor to the side as I wish to open my heart a bit to you and share some wisdom from an old fart who has paid a large price while dealing with health challenges, so here goes:

1.   Do not put your life on hold while you wait for the medical field to heal your infirmities. Throughout my "episodes" of bad health, I have learned the hard way that regardless of your condition in life, life goes on for you and for those most important to you. Personally, and I must admit regretfully, I missed out on some wonderful times and events that I chose not to attend due to my current "condition" all the while waiting for doctors to come up with an answer. Or, I would simply excuse myself by saying that I was not able to participate in certain events or activities because I didn't feel well. Now sometimes I really did feel like crap, and I would have been a burden had I participated. In those cases, of course I should not have done so. But there were other occasions when I simply decided not to go as it might have been a bit inconvenient to do so. Sometimes when I didn't feel so hot, I would get into the rut of a daily routine that was nothing more than a survival mode of just getting by with what I had to do for the day. So, I would go to work and do the minimum amount of work required, and then I would come home, sit in my easy chair and watch TV or lie down for a while. Then, my ever-patient wife would bring me dinner in my chair, and she would sit in the other chair while the TV was on so that we could spend some time together each day. I know for a fact that she would much rather have been doing something else, but it was my routine damn it, and she was either going to conform or do something else by herself! Perhaps I may just have been a little bit of a jerk — ya think? So, we pathetically spent many a night sitting together in our "His and Hers" recliners watching a movie re-run or television or sports show so that she could have the privilege of spending some time with me that day. I know that many a day and many a TV show or movie went by that she didn't like watching, but it was important to her that we spend time together. By the way, I have submitted my wife's name for sainthood. I am just waiting for the response to officially confirm her title. And when my wife would ask me if I wanted to go somewhere with her or do something with friends or family, I was reluctant to do so and use my current health condition as an excuse to stay home.

Now there were some days when I absolutely did not feel like doing anything. But, I found that with me, the excuses came more and more frequent and easier and easier to express, and I found myself home, alone, and living a hollow existence. Even worse than this was the fact that others—including our kids—began to notice a change in my personality. They found themselves avoiding me so that I would not be forced to do something with them when I "didn't feel good." They noticed that I became quieter and more anti-social, while becoming less jovial and less talkative. It hurts me to say that it took my kids telling me what my (so-called nagging) wife had already told me. The more that time passed, I found the rut getting deeper and deeper, while the excuses became easier and easier. So, if you find yourself in the rut of medical excuses and placing your precious life on hold until the doctors cure you and you bounce back to 100%, then kick yourself in the butt, climb out of the rut, and go on with your life. Don't miss out on one more precious day with those you love and who love you!

2. Do not underestimate the healing powers of a healthy lifestyle that includes exercise and proper nutrition. I have to be careful not to be a hypocrite here. I must disclose right now that my personal history is not unblemished when it comes to exercise and nutrition. This is a principle that I am still trying to have some consistency in following. And, even though I keep trying and trying to live a healthy lifestyle, I still fall way short and have to re-learn this principle over and over and over again. Even with the best intentions and attempting earnestly to recommit to start over each Monday (and boy is that a lot of Mondays!), I still end up slipping and following my favorite diet plan—the "see food" diet (which means that whatever I see, I eat). And in conjunction with this "see food" diet, I follow my personal exercise program of going on walks to the fridge and working out my arms by pulling my recliner lever and power lifting my spoon full of ice cream to my mouth. But, on those occasions in which I am eating a well-balanced diet, and I am getting some sort of exercise that gets my heart rate up for about a half hour a day, then (magically) I sleep better, and I have more energy to do so much more in a single day, and my disposition is greatly improved. I know that we have all heard these a thousand times, but there is absolutely no substitute for living a healthy lifestyle of diet and exercise. Whether you go to the gym or go for a walk, as long as you are getting some exercise, you will feel better. And, remember, this is not a diet book, but my advice is to eat right and eat healthy. If you are 40 years old or older, you know your own limitations on food. You know what you can eat and digest, and you know what types of food will kick back at you. So eat smart.

3.   **Do not become a prisoner to pain medications.** This is a big one for me! I know from personal experience that opiate pain medications are addictive. I also know that I personally have an "addiction gene" in my genetic makeup that gives me some challenges with impulsive behavior. This can be a very volatile combination. However, I also know that I have passed through some health issues that have required me to take these medications so that I can get through the day. The problem is that over time, your body builds up a resistance to the medications so that you need to take more and more pills to get the same pain relief. And while you're at it, after this resistance accumulates, it takes more and more pills for you to get that wonderful "buzz" from the opiates. The result is that over time, you end up getting hooked. I realize that this is

common knowledge, but just because everyone knows the hazards of dealing with opiates, that doesn't mean that we shouldn't openly and frequently talk about it. Coming from a guy who has been through three different pain management clinic treatments to step down off of opiates, I can tell you that it is important to think about and discuss this subject often. The point I am trying to make here is not just that pain medications are addictive. Pill addictions carry with them another issue that can be more destructive than the addiction factor alone.

The real bad part is that when you start counting pills every day and you start to panic when you get low and you have to contact your doctor several times a day as you start to run out— especially if your prescription is going to run out on a weekend when you are not able to contact your doctor—and suddenly you find yourself completely out of pills on a Saturday when you really start to freak out! Or, you start to plan your day completely around when you will be taking your next pill, and you push yourself and focus your thoughts on that next little hit. When you get to this point, your top priority is your next pill and your attention is continuously focused on just that one little pill. When this starts to happen, the pills have taken control of your life and you need to get some help and fast! Don't wait for your family or your kids to ask you what is wrong with you and why you are not as happy as you used to be and then they spend less and less time with you because they don't want to upset you. When this happens and when your pills take precedence over your wife or kids or work or anything else, then you have a problem and you need to get help now!

4. **Never forget the importance of close relationships.**
I am a firm believer that people who suffer from addictions or depression or even mental illness have a very powerful cure right at their fingertips. And this cure is free. The most effective form of treatment for overcoming addictions and other health issues is simply the power of love. This power is generated through the love that we share with our close friends and loved ones— especially our immediate family. When we find ourselves stuck in an addiction or other health challenge, and we recognize that we have people in our lives who love us and deeply care for our well-being, then it's like the proverbial light bulb goes on in our heads and we are suddenly grasped by an overwhelming desire to seek out whatever help we can get in order to get better!

I know many people who are very intelligent and educated on the risks of getting hooked on prescription drugs and yet because these people have alienated themselves from those whom they love by choosing to ignore their loving advice and continue to live a destructive lifestyle, they never seem to get better. This is because they have lost a strong enough reason to change and quit and seek help and get better. These people end up living a very shallow and bleak existence and end up very alone and sometimes confined to a bed either at home or at a medical institution. I am very familiar with others with the same level of education, yet they seek help and do whatever it takes to get over their addictions and destructive behavior because of a compelling motivation to get well in order to be with the ones they love. This compelling motivation is love. So, listen to the people who love you the most and seek help when they tell you that you have a problem. Do not be so selfish as to think that you know what's right for you better than they do and be so self-centered and self-destructive as to reject their loving advice and alienate yourself from your loved ones. If you do, you could end up very bitter, very alone, and maybe even very dead!

5. Do not allow frustration and discouragement to take hold of your happiness and positive state of mind and poison your outlook. I can sympathize with you better than most on this topic, and it is easier said than done isn't it? But don't you just hate it when you ask someone how he or she is doing and then you have to listen to a long list of problems? I know that for me, I will only ask this person how they are doing just once because with that type of response they have now been permanently labeled either Eeyore, or Hypochondriac, or both! Then, if I do come in contact with them in the future and believe me when I say that I do everything in my power to avoid them at all costs, I will purposely say "Good to see you," NOT "How are you doing?" I can only speak for myself here, but I do not want to ever be like that person who is constantly complaining about their health problems, because they are miserable, and misery seeks company.

I know that is it hard to be positive when you have suffered from pain for so long. And, even the most positive person gets tired of faking it long enough. However, I do believe that if you're not feeling very happy and you fake it, after a while, you feel a lot happier than if you just walk around all day like a walking billboard advertising miserableness. A very famous book (Dare I say the Bible?) talks about hypocrites who when they are fasting, walk around in public groaning from hunger pains and complaining about how hungry they are. And everyone around them knows that they are fasting and that they are miserable. The point is that they will get their recognition for fasting. I think that acting happy is like that. If we fake it long enough, then we will become it. So, like the song says, if you're happy and you know it, or even if you're not happy and you know it, fake a smile, or something like that.

I will never forget the little saying that goes something like this: I knew of a man who complained about his old, worn-out shoes until he saw a boy who had no feet. No matter how bad we are feeling or what health challenge we are going through, there is someone out there who is worse off than we are. But more than that, if we focus our efforts in helping out that someone else who is worse off than we are, and we take our minds off of our self and lose the self-pity by serving others, we will tend to forget our own problems by realizing that we aren't quite so bad off as we thought we were.

6.   Find some kind of release. For me, it has been to write about my challenges using humor. It is actually ironic, but I began writing this book as a way to deal with my health challenges. And, I started to share the more humorous adventures that I have shared here with others, including my friends and work associates and even my students. What I found out was this—not only did I find a good release from sharing these stories and focusing on their retelling in a humorous way, it also actually made me feel better. I do know a little about humor being a natural high by stimulating the production of endorphins, or happy hormones. I know through personal experience that this concept is true. So, as you deal with your health challenges, follow these four simple suggestions: 1. Always keep your sense of humor. 2. Try to find the humor in your own personal health history—I know that you can always find something funny about your own particular health story just as I have found in mine. 3. Find someone to share your funny story with then spare no humor when sharing it. And 4. Share it often and to a variety of audiences. It's amazing how much better you will feel. And, you will in turn, help others feel happier too! If we try hard enough, this could actually turn into an epidemic of enormous magnitude as we all spread this miraculous healing disease of humor!

7.   Maintain a positive outlook! Take your health into your own hands! Don't let your life pass you by while you wait for the doctor to "cure" you. I recognize that each person is different and that whenever you change your diet or exercise program, you should consult with your doctor if you have any concerns whatsoever. In my case, I decided that if was to get better, it was up to me to make the changes in my life to make it happen. So, I decided to implement what I call my "Poor Man's Wellness Program." The reason why I call it this is because my plan is very simple; it doesn't cost very much, and just about anyone can do it—anywhere, in whatever stage of life you find yourself, in different degrees of physical health, and on any kind of budget.

I am the first to admit that I have been on countless diet and exercise plans. And, I have had a fitness club membership for decades—literally. But, I am always breaking diets, I hate exercise programs and usually they end up hurting my back and knees and so they are short lived. And, as I said earlier, I am a school teacher and so my family lives on a limited budget. With that said, I have actually received some sound advice from my doctors, nutritionists, and diet counselors—oh yes, I have had a personal diet counselor that I reported to each week for my weigh-ins when I would wear as little as possible without being obscene in order to keep that damn scale from blurting out my actual weight. Then after weigh-in, I would hold counseling sessions where I would have to share my challenges and confess to my cheating. Heck, I sometimes I felt as if I were sitting in a confessional with the Pope himself and I had committed adultery, or that I was being interrogated by the FBI for making a bomb in my garage (I assure you that I have done neither.) I admit that I just hated to go to weekly weigh-ins, but they are the very reason why the diet worked so well. That is what kept me accountable—and being accountable is what makes a diet successful!

I have even been to pain management doctors who put me on pain therapy programs, including going for physical therapy, three times a week for six to eight weeks to learn proper stretching and exercises for my bad back and knees. Going through all these different attempts to improve my health and physical and psychological well-being, I have picked up some very good and practical tips that I have recently put into practice in my own life.

My "Poor Man's Wellness Program" program also takes into consideration that I am not a perfect and well-disciplined machine and that I will cheat and even take days off. And, I will even get a milkshake or eat a cookie now and then and I will not be dragged down to the depths of Hades by some dark, shadowy demon-like phantoms if I do slip and indulge now and then. If you are going to be successful in your own wellness program, then you must be flexible too.

Over the years of going to doctors, weight counselors, and physical therapists, I have learned some valuable advice to help me develop my own plan of wellness. By following my simple and flexible plan, my back feels better, I am losing weight, and

I am feeling younger and more energetic than I have in a very long time. So, I would like to share with you my low budget plan of a healthier lifestyle:

I. Take 40 minutes to 60 minutes a day to do some sort of aerobic exercise for half the time and then some sort of swimming the other half of the time. The best pain management doctor I ever visited told me that because I had a bad back and knees, I was limited in what kind of exercises I could do that were pain free. He then told me that what I needed was an exercise that was friction and impact pounding free. I told him that I used to jog, but I couldn't do that anymore and so now I liked stair-masters or elliptical machines. He told me that these exercises machines were a lot better, but I was still dealing with the weight of my own body putting pressure on my lower back and joints every time I took a step. He then told me that there is no body weight or body resistance when there is no gravity. I made some sarcastic remark about working out on a space station. He then reminded me that there is very little weight or body resistance in a swimming pool.

He then told me that if you were to take two of me, identical to each other, and one swam or did pool aerobics or even just treaded water on a regular basis, and the other person didn't, after ten years these two of me's would be completely different people health wise and even appearance wise-if in fact the one who never swam was still alive! That hit me lie a ton of bricks!

I first tried to go and swim at the pool at the fitness center. This works just fi ne and if you have a membership and perhaps you live in an apartment or somewhere that has cold winters, the local fitness center is great. Even if there is a local YMCA or public pool or community center, go to a local pool.

And, if you have warm summers, or if you live in California like I do where we have a nice climate all year round and you have a pool, then use your own pool. Or, if you don't have a nice pool and you live on a tight budget like I do, go to one of the big warehouse stores or department stores and buy a dough boy, an above ground pool, like we did. Ours is 12 feet in diameter and four feet deep. So, every day, I spend 20 minutes to a half hour swimming a breast stroke around the pool with a frequent switching of directions, or I just tread water by laying on my back and doing the frog kick of a back stroke and a forward breast stroke with my arms. This simple exercise done in a required space of 6 feet in diameter and four feet of water depth is a great exercise that virtually anyone can do! I am 6'5" tall and I can make it in 4 feet of water. I would bet that if I had to, or if I were smaller, I could even do it in 3 feet of water just fi ne. I even wear my little goggles and swimming ear plugs. I know that it sounds ridiculous, but hey, I'm in my backyard and even if my neighbors take a peek, they couldn't say anything because then I could have them arrested for being some kind of perverts or something! I have also found that during this time of swimming when I have the earplugs in and the goggles on and I am treading water, this is a great time for me to plan and organize my thoughts. It reduces my stress and I am able to think about and concentrate on important plans and ideas that I have going on. I am able to do so because I am eliminating all distractions—except for the occasional dead bug that floats by my goggles—and I can really focus my mind. I tell you that it really works!

In addition to my swimming or dog paddling or treading water, or whatever you want to call it, I then add 20 to 30 minutes of some sort of low-impact aerobics. You know what works for you and what doesn't. You also know what hurts and what doesn't, so my simple advice is this: if it hurts, don't do it. Find something that doesn't hurt and do that instead! I know—genius right? For me, I saved up some money and bought a nice elliptical machine. I use light settings and I don't listen to heavy metal so as to avoid a heart attack by escalated repetitions on the machine by keeping up with the beat of the music. A little bit of Phil Collins or the Eagles works great for me. You might enjoy your treadmill at home in front of the TV, if you can afford it and it works for you, then do that. If you can't afford some kind of aerobic machine, or if you don't have a machine, you could walk. My brother walks for 45 minutes a day. He loves it and he has done it for so long now, he couldn't go a day without going for a walk. It gets back to the old 21 days to create a habit idea.

If you can't afford some kind of aerobic machine, or if you have cold winters, join the new fad in indoor walking—go mall walking. Many people have converted to mall walking. You can go at your own pace, you are occupied while you walk by window shopping, the climate is always pleasant and controlled, you can mall walk with your friends and then enjoy a nice low-calorie treat to reward yourselves afterward, and best of all, you are walking in a very secure place. So, whatever you do and whatever is most comfortable and convenient for you—do it!

II. Eat a sensible diet. For me, I try to keep my caloric intake to 1500 to 1800 calories a day. Now remember that I have purchased food spending a hundred dollars a week or more from several different programs. What I learned was that you can get most of this food on your own at lower prices. For example, for breakfast, I have found that a diet that works for me is one and a half, or if I am real hungry, two instant oatmeals with a bit of fat free milk and some non-sugar sweetener works great. I learned that a package of oatmeal is offered for twice the price in those purchased food diet plans. If you don't like oatmeal, then find something for around 300 calories that you do like. Next, add some healthy snacks for midmorning like a snack sized can of fruit, or a low-fat yoghurt, or some fresh fruit and vegetables like pickles or radishes or carrots with some low-calorie dressing for dip. Then, for lunch, have a big salad and add whatever you like—within reason—that makes it taste good to you. I like to add a few slices of lean ham and sprinkle on some parmesan cheese. Now that we have some great tasting salad dressings in the local grocery stores, find one or two you like and pour them on your salad with a bit of self-discipline when you pour it. Or, you can find a good and simple frozen food meal that you can microwave that tastes pretty good. These are great for the office. If you are out of town, then try to use good judgment when you order. You know what is fattening and what isn't, so just do your best. Next, you need to have an afternoon snack or two. If you're like me, after I have had some salad or especially if I have had a bit of Chinese food, all it takes is one good fart and I am hungry again. So, if that happens, or if your lunch was light and you get hungry in the afternoon, have something on hand. Once again, fresh fruit or raw vegetables are perfect. I also like to take the edge off by eating some fat-free cottage cheese with some canned peaches or pears—packed in water of course! But if you're like me, I get kind of sick eating pickles or carrots all the time, and radishes give me bad breath—especially if they are dipped in low-cal ranch dressing. So, I love to have on hand some of those pre-packaged 100 calorie snacks that you can buy just about anywhere. They taste good and they are pretty satisfying. Buy one box that is salty and one that is sweet, as some days you are in the mood for one more than the other. For dinner, just eat sensibly. eat a variety of healthy breads or rice, with some fresh vegetables, and a smaller portion of meat—like 6 to 8 ounces. You can also find some great low-calorie meals in the frozen foods section of the local grocery store that are pretty good and that total less than 400 calories. These are great portion sizes and also very convenient if you are on the road, especially since most motels offer microwave ovens in their rooms.

Now comes the tough part of the day—evening time—you know, when the TV goes on. I know for a fact that when the TV comes on Lucifer comes out with his little demon friends to go around and poke us with their pitch forks filled with a devilish formula of potions formulated to make us ravishingly hungry! For most people—even me, I can do just fi ne all day until I sit down to watch TV at about eight or nine o'clock. It is then when my stomach begins to rumble, and my fingers start to twitch, and I find myself unconsciously rising up out of my recliner to head for the kitchen. This is the time when most of us take our diets by the neck, mercilessly shove them out the window, and thunder to the kitchen to snag whatever is sweet and gooey or buttery and salty, and we take our newly conquered booty back to our seat and start up our program again. Thank goodness for DVR! If this is the case, then we need to have some snacks on hand that can conquer our ravishing hunger and take away these long ago-programmed desires to graze at night.

For me personally, I love ice cream. I always have, and I always will. To subdue this never-ending night craving, I have some fat-free frozen yoghurt of my favorite flavors in the freezer, and I force myself to not put any toppings on it, and I use a regular bowl instead of a mixing bowl that in my cupboard says ice cream and breakfast cereal bowl all over it! Or, I will make a home-made smoothie with a yoghurt base and some fresh fruit with a little frozen yoghurt or fat free milk to give it a creamy base. You can also buy some smoothie mixes in a variety of flavors if you wish. Or, you could also get those microwavable smart popcorns that come in 100 calorie packages.

If you're like me and my wife, and if you're cheap like us, you can even pre-pop these and take them to the movies with you. With the new gigantic purses out there today, it is very easy to smuggle in your favorite snacks to avoid the popcorn with extra dripping butter added at the half way mark and then again on the top of the container—for true movie popcorn connoisseurs like I am. And, since you are breaking your diet that night only, you buy a half-pound bag of candy to go along with it. And you end up actually gaining more weight in that one night alone than the total weight of the junk food that you just ate! So, what will it be, two thousand calories at the movies or 200? The choice is yours. And you can decide the 200 calories and take in a pre-packaged sweet snack and a 100-calorie pre-popped popcorn and still enjoy the movie and take away the hunger pangs while you're at it.

The absolute critical factor for this diet to work is to gut it out the first week—especially the first three days. What I mean is that when we diet, our body kind of rebels in a defensive mode because we are ripping away the sugar, fats and starches that we are used to eating. We may even get headaches besides those awful stomach pangs. So during the first three days of the diet, make sure that you keep yourself busy and when you are suffering, and oh my friends how you will suffer, make sure that you have some low-calorie snacks on hand like pickles or carrots or 100-calorie snack bags or even some extra frozen yoghurt or fruit or even hot chocolate or coffee or tea. (I have found that hot drinks tend to make you feel satisfied when you are hungry.) If you make it past the first three or four days, the body has pretty well adjusted and your new nutrition plan will become easier. One critical thought: I have learned from years of experience to listen to your body when it talks to you. The human body is an amazing machine and if it needs something, it will let you know—kind of like your car. So, if you feel hungry, eat a bit more. If your body is craving some carbs, then make a reasonable sandwich. If you listen to your body and give it what it asks for, it won't scream at you so much when it is deprived of the garbage that it is used to eating.

III. Now that you have the exercise and diet taken care of, you can really help yourself by making yourself accountable. When I was paying 100 dollars a week and I was seeing my personal weight counselor, the most compelling reason why I didn't cheat, and I followed the program to the letter was that I did not want to face my counselor if I had cheated. She would know that I had cheated because during our little weigh-in, she would record my weight and that damn scale would never cover for me or even stretch the truth, even just a little bit, and I would be betrayed every time. And so, if you can have a weekly weigh-in with someone you trust, and you are comfortable with them, then do it. In fact, if you two make a contest out of it and you both hold weekly weigh-ins together as a competition with a nice prize going to the winner—even better! If not, then have your own weekly weigh-in and record your weight once a week. In fact, our weight fluctuates from day to day and so don't weigh yourself every day.

Only weigh yourself once a week and write it down.

Speaking of writing it down, I also learned from these programs that you should plan your meals daily and write down what you eat every day and keep that in the same little journal or notebook where you write down your weight. For me personally, I write down the calories I eat for each meal and every snack. And at the end of the day, I plan what I eat and what I snack on to stay at about 1500 to 1800 calories. Each person's metabolism is different, and I am no doctor, so you need to consult your doctor as to what your individual calorie intake should be. I have found that for me—and I am a big guy—that 1500 to 1800 calories of the right foods are okay for me. It is critical for all of us to not starve ourselves. If we do, then our brain and body think that we are starving and then they begin the shutdown procedures that store fat and stop us from burning calories and losing weight. So, the key is to eat enough to never be hungry and give us the energy we need to get through the day and feel good. When we feel good, we are happy. There is no substitute for this simple philosophy.

IV. The last key component to this or any diet and exercise program is to remember that you are not a machine and that you will have some days when you slip or screw up and don't do any exercise and you pig out. Heck, no one is perfect and we all have our weaknesses and days when we just say, "screw it" and pig out. Okay, we do it and it happens—so what. In fact, sometimes it is great to treat yourself when you are doing well and in the groove of losing weight and exercising. Go ahead and treat yourself every once in a while — just don't do it very often and be smart about it. If you are eating out or traveling, try to exercise and eat right as best you can. Then, get back to your regular routine as soon as you can. Remember it is said or at least I have heard research that says that it takes about 21 days to form a habit, and about a week or a bit less to break one. So, create habits for yourself with regards to fitness and nutrition and don't break them. You can bend them once in a while, but don't break them. Diet and exercise can be enjoyable. They don't have to be torture. If they are unpleasant for you, then they won't work because you won't like what you are doing, and you will find excuses to stop. But if you enjoy your individual diet and exercise plan, then you are more likely to stick with it and have a happier and healthier life! I truly believe the wise saying about food: We eat to live, not live to eat. If you think about this as a guideline for self-control with regard to eating habits, it is quite profound.

My crazy journey through this labyrinth of health challenges and perhaps somewhat unique encounters with the medical community have led me down a path that will stop for now at a crossroads I now face that will take me into the stages of later adulthood. So far, my sojourn has taken me through some turbulent, yet comical episodes. The path that lies before me now will certainly be nothing less than incredible. The attitude with which I face it will greatly determine the outcome.

And so as I approach the wall that leads me into my next adventure, I ask you to reflect, along with me, this final consideration: When we stick our heads through this hole in the wall we call life, what we choose to see on the other side as we open our eyes is the defining force by which we will deal with life's little bumps and bruises. As for me, I will do it with a smile   on   my   face,   and   humor   in   my   heart.

Chapter 10
As a Dog Returns to Its Vomit…

"As a dog returns to his vomit, so a fool repeats his folly" is an aphorism which appears in the Book of Proverbs in the Bible — Proverbs 26:11. Now I realize that this book hopefully is not my folly. With that said, I am compelled to return to my book and add another chapter.

Eight years have passed since I wrote the second edition of this book. And as my fate might have it, I have also passed through some noteworthy medical events that must be brought forth into my health's proverbial light of day. I owe it to you – the reader of my medical history – no matter how many or how few you are – to divulge the events of these past eight years. After all, what would Back to the Future be like if there were no film number three? Can you possibly imagine never knowing the rest of the story? Our lives would be void of the enriching saga that tells of Dr. Emmet Brown's traveling back to the wild west to face the notorious outlaw Buford "Mad Dog" Tannen. Imagine what life would be like if for some bizarre series of events, season eight of Game of Thrones were to be canceled in mid-season?

Okay, I suppose that I am a bit presumptuous, nay, to some even blasphemous to put my book in the same category as these two iconic, cinematic tales. But for me, as I face the stark reality of turning sixty years old this year, I am constrained to add another chapter. Anything after this, just as a Back to the Future Four or Game of Thrones season 9, will be a bonus. For in this season or sequel of the annals of my Aesculapian (meaning health or medical, but sort of sounds like a word young maester Sam might say as he studies the ancient medical records for a possible cure for the dreaded greyscale) history, I have now traveled beyond the DeLorean–esque journeyings through the milestones of knee replacements on both knees, detached retinas on both eyes and last but in no way least, a Thrones-sounding, yet actual modern medical malady known as Hammertoe!

Knee Replacement

As I delve into the "Dark Side" forces of knee replacement, I must warn you that this tremendous medical advancement that literally changes your life by eliminating the anguish of chronic knee pain and its accompanying inability to literally walk from any point A to point B, is in reality best described as a barbaric, medieval Bastard Executioner style procedure, that utilizes power tools that could be found at your local Home Depot medical isle!

Before I scare you away from considering this procedure, let me just say that having this procedure on both knees literally changed my life! I went from barely being able to walk from my parked car to my high school classroom, to now being able to perform daily 45-minute workouts on the elliptical machine without suffering from any subsequent knee pain or joint stiffness (with the aid of a 20-minute icing for my chronic back pain afterward!). However, because I made the mistake of watching the video of the procedure given me by my doctor, (Spoiler Alert – Do NOT watch the video until after you have had both knees replaced!) I discovered that this procedure includes the use of drills, saws, files, sanders, hammers, and some industrial strength glue!

Never-the-less, my new titanium knee joints are incredibly strong and resilient, and their shelf life is estimated to be – well, let's just say that if it's good enough for The Terminator, then it's good enough for me!

HOWEVER...

This type of surgery is not all cupcakes and lollipops! This is not one of those surgeries where you are given some pain pills, then sent home to prop your knee up with a pillow and settle in to your recliner to catch up on all the great TV miniseries and cable shows you have not yet had the time to watch, while sipping on your favorite beverage and munching on a bag of chips – all while your knee magically heals itself!

Oh no you don't!

Recovery from this procedure is anything but easy! If I could compare the discomfort and pain level of this procedure – at least for the first two weeks – to let's say an experience that the readers could better relate to...let me think...I would have to say something like...let's see...A wild grizzly bear attack where the beast chomps down on your knee joint, then shakes his head from side to side, with your knee in his mouth. If the reader can't relate to that then, um, how about, oh yeah! We just had Shark Week on TV! And there were these Great Whites playing volleyball with seals! Yes, that should do it! Picture that volleyball game with your knee as the ball!

Now I must clarify here that I had one knee done, then, six months later, I had my other knee replacement surgery. I know of some poor fools – including my very own brother, and my mother-in-law (Mom if you are reading this, I am not calling you a fool! In fact, you are a kind, considerate and very bright humanitarian to whom I look up to and for whom I have a great deal of respect) – who had both knees done at the same time! How terrible would that be? How could you recover? How could you ever walk? One of the keys to complete recovery from this surgery is to get up and walk on the same day of the surgery! How in thee hell does one get up and walk when both knees have been sliced open and have been more brutalized than one of the poor unsuspecting victims of the movie "Saw?" I have so much respect for those out there who had to pass through this Job-like trial. Fortunately for me, and I think for most knee replacement patients these days, doctors now do one knee at a time, as it should be.

To understand the pain level, all I need to tell you is that before you go under the power tools, the anesthesiologist comes in for a little visit. And during that visit, he or she, but in my case he, tells you that because of the aggressiveness of the procedure – you know – when the grizzly has chomped down and is flailing your limb about as if it were a twig – recommends that you get general anesthetic to make sure that you are in La-La Land, and ALSO that you have a spinal block, so that when you awake from anesthetic, the spinal block slowly wears off so that you gradually get used to the pain that will inevitably rise from a pain level of one, all the way up to, about uh...let's see...oh yeah, TO A GOOGLE!

Okay, so you have woken up, the spinal tap has worn off and you have just had a hospital popsicle – ice chips while imagining that a fruity flavoring has been added – and you have had a nice injection of dilauded (the wonder painkiller), the physical therapist comes in for a visit. I must warn you that when this individual enters the room, they smile at you, ask how you are doing, ask how much pain you are in, and overall appear to be your friend. But beware my friend, for you would no more call this individual your friend than adapt that grizzly to replace your house cat that just passed away! Or, fill your swimming pool with saltwater and invite those Great Whites over for a swim party and play volleyball – with you as the ball! The physical therapist, whom I will refer to here on out as Lucifer Incarnate, came into my room and pretended to care about my pain level and act as if she was concerned about how I was doing. Then, she asked me to inch my way over to the side of the bed. She wrinkled her eye brows and turned the edges of her mouth downward in an expression of shared pain and concern, while on the inside, she put on a party hat and blew into a noise-maker, while swimming in a sea of balloons! Her eager anticipation of my approach to the edge of the bed caused a slight line of liquid drool to escape her lips and wind its way down the edge of her chin.

Once I had reached the edge of the bed, Little Miss L.I. instructed me to rotate my hips in a way to bring my operated on wrapped leg out over the bed, so that the recently power tool – repaired appendage, looking like the remains of a sky-scraper crane after going through a category five hurricane, in all its vulnerability, would be in a better position to be slowly lowered down to the floor. Be mindful that once the naked and afraid XXXL leg was looming over the side of the bed cliff, I had no control to keep it there! So, my leg – that if could sing would be booming out its own rendition of Tom Petty and the Heartbreakers' Free Fallin' – dropped to the icy floor of what I now realized was no hospital room at all, but what had revealed itself in a painkiller induced, hallucinogenic state, to be a medieval torture chamber!

Once the rockets red glare, and the bombs bursting in air stopped flashing before my eyes and my vision began to clear, and the jolts of pain shooting from my knee to the pain center of my brain had subdued, and I had stopped my listless blubbering, I took several deep breaths and whispered a question. Well, at least I tried to ask the question, and it's true that my mouth was open, and my lips were moving, but the only sounds that came forth out of my mouth were the indistinguishable hissing sounds of a catatonic psyche ward lunatic!

The amazing thing of it all was that Lucifer understood exactly what I was saying. She responded without hesitation and complete confidence and told me that I was doing great and that yes, the next step in my rehab from hell was for me to grasp the handgrips on either side of the walker, which she had so nonchalantly placed in front of me – like the captain of a firing squad handing the live round of ammunition to the randomly selected shooter! Her next instructions were spoken in such a way as if she were asking of me nothing more than winking an eye or shaking her hand but would be better compared to her demanding that I walk the plank over shark-infested waters or put on some size fifteen ballet shoes and dance the Nutcracker! She instructed me to sand up! Just stand up! Sure! That's all! No Problem! There's nothing to it! Que Sera, Sera, and These Are a Few of My Favorite Things, and Just a Spoon Full of Sugar Helps the Medicine Go Down!

Because I was raised by a loving mother, and I was taught by my father to always show the respect to women that they deserve, and even though this was no ordinary woman – nay, and dare I pose the question asking if she was even human at all, I did as she said and I gripped the sides of that walker likened to Arthur grasping that sword in the stone. Then, placing my good foot directly in front of me and leaning forward with all my might as if I were Jack Dawson holding onto Rose Dewitt over the front edge of the Titanic, I smiled as the salty breeze of the treacherous cafeteria sea struck my face. Placing more upper body weight on my hands and shaking like Jack as he held on to his beloved Rose while treading the icy waters off Newfoundland, I began to stand. Several times, my leg began to buckle but knowing that life will go on and on, I persevered! Even though I wanted to give up and give in to the frigid Pacific waters of despair, I continued to lift my body off the bed until I stood – upright and erect – and quivering like a newborn horse standing and taking its first step, I took mine! Triumphant, I stood with the pride of an Olympic champion! I had done it! If looks could speak, my gaze upon the physical therapist would remind one of Wyatt Earp as he looked down the barrel of his Smith and Wesson and fired the mortally wounding round at the pathetic Billy Clanton, who was no match for the likes of the greatest lawman ever to wear a badge in the notorious old west!

I had completed my task and was about to sit back down and treat myself to a victorious reward for my efforts with the only safe hospital food I have ever known – chocolate pudding – when the beast from the underworld of rehab spoke once more! As the poisonous spittle spewed out of her mouth, mixed with her toxic terminologies of total trepidation, her words would shake me to the core of my very being! The audacity of this demon instructed me now to walk to the bathroom to see if I can make it on my own to the toilet, in order to pacify any further concerns among the nursing staff who were already on 24-7, DEFCON 1, Bedpan Call of Doodie!

I could see the beast's lip quiver after giving me the instructions to take this trek – a voyage that seemed to me at the time to be no more possible than Captain Hook hoofing it from California to the Klondike! She tilted her head like a zombie eye-balling an unsuspecting pedestrian, sizing him up for its next tasty meal! I could tell that she was hungry to watch my agonizing walk; her eyes widened like a child entering the Holiday-ornamented family room on Christmas morning!

My wife was in the room, so I knew that when I started my pilgrimage to the sacred porcelain palace, I could not deviate from the path long enough to bludgeon the zombie to death using my only weapon of choice – the very walker she had given me! I had no choice but to comply with the death wish – my only consolation was that I would in fact, be urinating the natural, God-given way of doing the deed, instead of requiring the use of another medieval torture device – the notorious catheter tube!

And so, with the aid of the walker, the encouragement of my wife and the incentive of mocking my torturer, I made the agonizing pilgrimage – step by painstaking step! With my new titanium device attached to my mangled, power tool ravaged flesh and bone, I could feel the thu-thump of my heartbeat depicted as only Edgar Allen Poe could describe in his legendary tale, "The Tell-Tale Heart." As the story goes, the sound of the heartbeat of the murdered old man gets louder and louder in the killer's mind, until he goes mad and confesses his crime. In my case, I must admit that I had a compelling urge to "off" the hag, dismember her body parts and place them under the floorboards of the infirmary! None-the-less, I endured the walk – step by agonizing step – and made it to the throne room, where I paid a pittance of liquid ransom.

At this point, I began to see stars. I am confident that the stars appeared as a result of both the painstaking walk and how hard I had to push to urinate. You see, when a knee replacement surgery is performed, the patient (in this case – me) is catheterized. Then, once I was in the recovery room and fortunately while the spinal block is still in effect, the catheter is removed. However, even with the tube removed, there still remains a considerable amount of inflamed tissue in the pipes! That's like saying that there was a little dust kicked up when Mount Saint Helens erupted! So, when I relieved myself, it was both effortful and painful.

After completing my assigned task, I about faced and began my long trek back to the welcoming arms of my bed, which beckoned my rear end ever homeward with the compelling force of a hard-boiled egg getting sucked back into a coke bottle with a match inside. The most difficult aspect of returning to the bed was to not go so fast as to wipe out on the homeward path. Thus, with focused concentration, I was able to clip-clop the walker legs back to the bed where I sat back down to the ecstatic relief of arriving back at my very own little safe place! The welcoming relief of the mattress felt like I had just returned home from escaping the hard labor work camp of a third world militant regime!

You may wonder why the explanation of my first post-op steps has taken up several pages. I would respond by asking if you would have been satisfied with a quick tweet saying, "First Step" from Neil Armstrong after taking mankind's historic first walk on the moon! My in-depth details may appear to you to be an exaggeration, but until you have passed through this ordeal yourself, you cannot judge my description of this extraordinary event in one's medical history.

I spent the rest of my first and only night at the hospital in the bliss of laying on my bed and enjoying getting loaded up on pain meds and a milkshake, which was snuck in by my wife.

The following morning, the physical therapist returned for round two. This time, she had brought with her a prop of her trade, made of wood. Would you like to guess what she brought? No, it was not a pillory (stockade), nor the wooden hydro-powered torture device from the Princess Bride's Pit of Despair. It appeared harmless enough – just a few boards nailed together to make two steps, but the Wicked Witch of the West (west hospital wing, that is) had located the torture device out in the hallway, so that I would have to use my four-legged walking device, with two wheels and two tennis balls on the front posts used for traction, to navigate my way out of the hospital room and into the hallway. Then, I would have to continue, step by agonizing step, until I arrived at this next challenging obstacle which stood in the way of my recovery process. At the time, you might just as well have told me to navigate the great Amazon River in a kayak, then climb Mount Everest!

However, by now, after reading most of this book, you realize that I have faced as many of these death-defying surgeries and medical procedures as Evel Knievel faced cars, busses, 18-wheelers and Grand Canyons! And so, I complied with the orders of my WWII concentration camp commandant, and with hands on walker, I commenced on my journey from my bedside to the great hallway. I again went through the procedure of standing at my bedside with the assistance of my new four-legged best friend. Once I stood, I had to wait to allow the blood back into my head and body, which had dropped down to my knee so fast, it was as if my blood had taken a free-fall from 20,000 feet! Then, I began my cloppity-clop, step-limp synchronized stroll toward the hallway. This was about as synchronized as Walmart shoppers on Black Friday, when they open their doors for door-buster sales of everything from small appliances and TV's to fidget spinners!

Never-the-less, I took my time to make sure that my legs were well within the walls of Fido (my new four-legged aluminum friend), before I took each painstaking new step. As I looked at the physical therapist, it seemed as if she were wide-eyed and drooling – just hoping for a big wipe out – like a circling vulture waiting for the poor lost soul in the middle of a desolate desert to drop dead from heat exhaustion!

Yet even though my legs wobbled a few times, causing the big bad buzzard to twitch with anticipated delight, I stayed upright, making my way out into the hall until I had approached the steps up to the gallows of my worst nightmare. Next, Mrs. Satan told me that she was going to take the walker away from me and hand me my cane, since I could not use the walker to climb the wooden Everest. I cursed at her under my breath, yet I knew that I had to be prematurely weaned off of my aluminum binkie in order to climb the steps. Once my wife and a nurse were positioned on either side of me as my spotters, the beast-ess stripped me of my walker and replaced it with my cane. That must be like the ordeal a kid goes through when mom and dad take away their security blankie and replace it with a Disney character night light. The concept sounds good, but from the kid's point of view, he got totally screwed on that deal!

At this point, I was taught a simple chant: "Lead with the good leg going up, and with the bad leg going down." And although this sounds easy, once you start the process, and keep in mind that your leg has just gone through a trauma best compared to stepping on a land-mine, made by a deranged pyro-technic bomb maker from ISIS, you are bound to experience (p)fi, which is the mathematic formula that signifies pain to the power of f'ing infinity!

And so, I faced that first step like the first step out of an airplane at 10,000 feet on my very first sky-diving experience. As I took the first step, a small amount of pee escaped onto my undies – just as would certainly happen on both sides of my shorts if I ever jumped out of an airplane! My legs wobbled, and my spotters tightened their grips on my forearms. As I straightened my good leg and lifted my heavily-bandaged leg to the first of the two steps, I exhaled a breath of relief – only the air of relief that had escaped me exited out of my backside instead. I excused myself then taking a moment to regain my balance and some sense of stability, I boldly took the next (and last) step up. I made it! I started to raise my hands like Rocky Balboa as he reached the top step in victory, but I quickly bright them back down once I realized that I am really not like Rocky at all, but more like Methuselah of Biblical times, who was the oldest man on record at 969 years old at the time of his death!

I had made the trek up the wooden mount Sanai, and now I would have to go back down. In mountain climbing, 80% of all accidents occur on the way down, and in my mind, I just knew that this percentage was about ready to go up by one climber! And yet, with the aid of my spotters and my trusty cane, I made my way back down the biggest two-step of my life! (Well actually, there was this time down in Mexico when I ate a bad shrimp taco, but other than that...) And once I was back on solid ground (in my mind, I bent over and kissed the soil of my homeland), I was given back my aluminum binkie and made my way back to the bed. I made this trip in record time because I knew that there was an awesome award waiting for me once I was back on the bed. No, it wasn't a Frosty from Wendy's! Nope! It wasn't a large DQ Blizzard! I was going to get my next injection of pain medication!

On this, the second day, I was to be released to go home and convalesce – but convalesce was not the right word to describe my continued rehabilitation once I got home. I think a better descriptive word would be affliction, or tribulation or better yet – excruciation! I was not sent home to elevate my knee in my favorite recliner and watch all the re-runs and every cable series that I had not yet had the chance to watch while eating bon-bons and sipping on fruit smoothies! On second thought, I could sit in my favorite recliner, elevate my knee and watch re-runs and cable TV series while eating bon-bons and drinking smoothies, but every couple of hours, I had to do a series of "exercises," including taking laps around our first floor, and also a series of tormentuous (I don't think that is an actual word, but it is the best adjective I can think of) forced bending and straightening the knee exercises that were both difficult to do correctly and gritting-your-teeth-with-spittle-coming-out painful!

I must say that looking back on these exercises, because I did them more frequently, and I did more "reps" than instructed, the result was that my knee healed completely! As a result of doing the extra work, I now have a full range of motion with zero pain! And, because my legs are now straight, I walk with much better posture resulting in less back pain! I will always have to endure the symptoms of chronic back pain, but it is significantly better now that I no longer imitate the Leaning Tower of Pisa when I stand up!

Another thing that helped my healing process immensely was this icing contraption that my doctor gave me, called a Cryotherapy Arctic Ice Cold Water Therapy System. This contraption actually circulated ice water from a bucket of ice and water through a pad that circled my knee, providing me with soothing ice therapy after every series of exercises. It was like giving my knee a Blizzard after every workout! Just like the Co-eds where I went to college! I will never forget going to get a cone at 31 Flavors, only to wait in line behind a bunch of rather hefty college girls who had jogged there for a little nightcap! To this day, I could never figure that one out!

Once I went home, and after several weeks, my doctor referred me to attend two sessions a week of physical therapy at a rehabilitation facility, with the equipment and facilities for proper and complete rehab. My first day there was rather eye-opening, for it was there I came to the stark reality that I was getting old! As soon as I entered the room and began my treatment with a trained kinesiologist, I realized that I was surrounded by senior citizens! At first, I thought I must have gone to the wrong facility! And for a brief moment, I actually thought I had passed through the veil of death! I wanted to put a baseball cap on to cover my hair that had not yet turned a frosty white! However, after I while, I got used to my new surroundings and found my new work-out buddies to be very alive, and all sharing a very down-to-earth and humorous perspective of life and health and working toward the same objective of getting stronger – just like I had.

I must recommend that all who go through a knee replacement take full advantage of this type of facility. There is no way that one can properly rehabilitate a replaced knee joint without going through this six-week program! So, get the referral and as Nike has instructed us, "Do it!"

Moving forward in time about six months, once my first knee was recovered, I had my other knee replacement surgery. I will say that both the pain I experienced on this second go-round was more intense, and the rehab took longer and was more painful than the first. This may not be the case for any of you facing double knee-replacement, but it was with me. I think that part of the problem was that I had significant knee surgery during high school forty years ago, when this knee was surgically repaired. Well, you could call it surgery, just like the unique and bizarre surgical/medical procedures from the medieval era. Here are a few of my favorites that were actually performed back in the day:

Here is a description of the treatment of kidney stones: "If there is a stone in the bladder make sure of it as follows: have a strong person sit on a bench, his feet on a stool; the patient sits on his lap, legs bound to his neck with a bandage, or steadied on the shoulders of the assistants. The physician stands before the patient and inserts two fingers of his right hand into the anus, pressing with his left fist over the patient's pubes. With his fingers engaging the bladder from above, let him work over all of it. If he finds a hard, firm pellet it is a stone in the bladder... If you want to extract the stone, precede it with light diet and fasting for two days beforehand. On the third day, ... locate the stone, bring it to the neck of the bladder; there, at the entrance, with two fingers above the anus incise lengthwise with an instrument and extract the stone." Sounds like a deranged quarterback taking a hiked "ball" from a confused, submissive center! "Set...Hike!"

Another infamous practice was Blood-Letting. Physicians in the Middle Ages believed that most human illnesses were the result of excess fluid in the body (called humour). The cure was removing excess fluid by taking large amounts of blood out of the body. Two of the main methods of bloodletting were leeching and venesection.

In leeching, the physician attached a leech, a blood-sucking worm, to the patient, probably on that part of the body most severely affected by the patient's condition. The worms would suck off a quantity of blood before falling off. Escargot anyone?

Venesection was the direct opening of a vein, generally on the inside of the arm, for the draining of a substantial quantity of blood. The tool used for venesection was the fleam, a narrow half-inch long blade, which penetrates the vein, and leaves a small wound. The blood ran into a bowl, which was used to measure the amount of blood taken.

Monks in various monasteries had regular bloodletting treatments – whether they were sick or not – as a means of keeping good health. They had to be excused from regular duties for several days while they recovered. No kidding!!! Hey! Brother Alfred! I need a few days off because I cannot feel my legs! I just hope they never confused a venesectomy with a vasectomy! Yikes!

A third and final curious medical practice of the medieval period was known as *"Clysters,"* a method of injecting medicines into the anus. The medieval version of the enema was known as the clyster, which is really an instrument for injecting fluids into the body through the anus. The clyster was a long metallic tube with a cupped end, into which the medicinal fluid was poured. The other end, a dull point, which was drilled with several small holes, was inserted into the anus. Fluids were poured in and a plunger was used to inject the fluids into the colon area, using a pumping action.

The most common fluid used was lukewarm water, though occasionally medical concoctions, such as thinned boar's bile or vinegar, were used.
In the 16th and 17th centuries, the medieval clyster was replaced by the more common bulb syringe. In France, the treatment became quite fashionable. King Louis XIV had over 2,000 enemas during his reign, sometimes holding court while the ceremony progressed! No wonder King Louie liked to wear tights! As the classic song of the great movie, Robin Hood, Men in Tights so eloquently expresses, "We're men! We're men in tights – tight tights!"
Anyway, my point is that since I had had extensive surgery on this second knee over 40 years ago, which was performed prior to orthoscopic practices common today, this knee had atrophied more than the first, causing its own unique pattern of post-op healing. Thus, this second knee took longer, and required more extensive therapy sessions than did the first. This is not to insinuate that others who have both knees replaced will pass through similar results. Who knows, you just might need to have a few "Clysters" in your healing process!
My final bit of advice is this: when you are in your recovery period, follow the directions of your team of doctors and therapists! Do the work – even though it hurts, and don't stop until you have the maximum amount of flexibility your knee

will achieve based on your own unique set of circumstances. By the way, I have heard the surgical staff say that if you do not reach a full range of motion on your own, they will actually take you back to the hospital, put you under general anesthetic, and force straighten, or force bend your knee joint until you do! So, do the work on your own terms!

One more suggestion I can give you refers to the occasion when the doctors first take off your bandages, revealing what appears to be a cadaver leg after several hundred practice repairs. Your leg will be black and blue, and there will be a fifteen-inch bloodied line going down your leg stapled with about twenty-five staples! So, when you take a peek at the carnage for the first time, you may want to take a pain pill about a half hour before, so that even though it looks horrendous, you won't seem to mind much! Be sure to take a picture of your leg's transformation to Transylvania while you're at it, so you can Tweet it to all your friends and family. The picture is sure to gross-out your friends and for family members, once they see the picture, they will be so much more sympathetic and extend the time they will show you gestures of sympathy – like cakes and pastries and cookies and meals, etc.

So, hang in there and do the work, use the ice, take full advantage of pain medication (but don't get hooked!), and just plain survive for the first two weeks. After that, the rest of your rehabilitation is all downhill!

Detached Retinas

The summer of 2016 was going to be one for the family vacation record books. Almost our entire family was finally going to vacation in Orlando Florida and do the whole theme park experience. My wife and I had been looking forward to spending time with our grandkids at Disney World, Epcot,

Universal Florida and even an alligator farm! And even though I had my knee replacement surgery only five weeks before, we were planning on getting me a wheelchair, which to the ecstasy of our kids, would get us up in the front of the lines!

My orthopedic surgeon had told me that I was supposed to wait eight weeks before flying, to avoid any possible blood clots, but I figured that five weeks was close enough – wasn't it? Well, if you were to ask God or Karma if five weeks were enough for me, the answer, I guess, was a resounding NO!

Because with less than a week to go until we got on the plane to Florida, I woke up with an eye problem! Only this problem could be compared to saying that you are having car problems, like your car won't start, when in actuality, the car had been totaled and was sitting in a salvage yard, with the only undamaged parts available for sale being the floor mats!

My problem was that I could see, but only in half of my field of vision.in one eye. Looking through the other half of that eye's field of vision was like looking through a dark cloud of smoke! I must say that this was a very unsettling experience! It sort of reminded me of when I had Lasik surgery done on my eyes when just before the doctor starts to laser away some eye lens tissue – which by the way I could smell, he slices open the eye and opens it up like a can of tuna! And when that happens, and he peels back the lid, your vision disappears so that even though your eye is open, all you see is black nothing!

Once I realized that it wasn't a cloudy contact lens, or a big booger covering my eye, I called the ophthalmologist and they had me come right down! It must have been pretty bad for me to get an immediate appointment – I thought that you had to have a major limb hanging by a thread of skin for that to happen!

However, the appointment-making staff messed up and mistakenly made my appointment with an eye doctor where I would usually go to get my annual vision checked for vision prescriptions. When I met with him, I was told that I needed to see a specialist and to call a nurse hotline, where I could get a pre-diagnosis over the phone. This is supposedly reserved for patients with serious conditions. So, I gave her a call. She told me that I would be getting a call from an eye doctor within two hours and if I didn't, I was to go to the ER. In my 59 and ¾ years of life, I have only been told that once before and that was when my doctor called me in the middle of teaching my high school class, when after getting my bloodwork results, he called and told me that he thought I was having a heart attack! (It ended up that my heart was fine, but my gall bladder was infected and gangrenous, so my bloodwork was all messed up!)

Well, I didn't get the call, so I went to the ER and just as I was checking in, I got the call on my cell phone and they said the specialist could see me in a half hour. His office was located in an adjacent building. So, I walked to the next-door building and checked in. In about five minutes, I was called back to see the doctor. Talk about fast service! I must say that I was both relieved and grateful to be seen so quickly, since all the while I was looking through that cloud in my eye and it wasn't getting any better!

So, he checked my sight with the letters he could possibly flash onto the wall. I guess that my looking at those huge letters could be compared to me standing fifty feet in front of the

Hollywood sign on the hill above movie town! And even though these same letters can practically be seen from space, all I could make out was a big white smudge! I was told that my vision in that eye was 20-4000, in other words, I was blind in the eye. He got out the bright flashlight and looked inside my eye and quickly identified my problem as a detached retina. He asked me a series of questions to see if I had experienced any trauma lately – a head injury, or physical exertion beyond my ordinary activities. All I could think of is that I sleep hard and sometimes I am constipated, but I did not see how poop could cause my eye to get a blow-out!

Anyway, he told me that the gel inside my eye had cracked due to age and being far-sighted as I was (That elongates the eyeball), some fluid had entered the crack and seeped in between the lining of my eye and my retina, causing it to detach.

As he continued to treat my condition, his next step was to inject my eye with a bubble of gas. The gas pressurized my eye, forcing the torn portion of my retina back toward the lining of the eye and keeping constant pressure on the retina to help it re-attach itself. The gas bubble would remain in my eye for about a month, after which time it would dissipate on its own and disappear from my view. But for the time being, as I looked straight ahead, I was literally looking through a big bubble!

After the bubble injection, the ophthalmology department scheduled me for surgery the next morning. The doctor told me to stay in a position with my head pointing down as much as possible, allowing the bubble to place constant pressure on the retina. He also told me to sleep on my side with my head pointed down. This instruction sort of worried me since I really never thought about the position of my head while sleeping, and I was not given a head alarm that would sound off every time my head would move into an upright position during sleep! I went to sleep repeating to myself over and over a chant to keep my face pointing in a downward position.

In our household, prayer is something that is done regularly. On this night, I was hoping that my standing with the Big Guy upstairs was solid! We called on a few favors that night to be sure, as I did not want to have eye surgery!

The next morning, I awoke to discover that amazingly enough, the bubble had done some good and my vision had cleared considerably. My wife drove me to the doctor's office and I must admit, thinking about eye surgery made me very nervous. After I was checked in, the doctor tested my vision in the cloudy eye. It had improved to 20 – 400! And, when the doctor examined my retina, it appeared that the retina had re-attached almost completely! The doctor said there was no need for surgery, to keep up with the head positioning, and to come back in two days, when he would perform a laser procedure and also possibly freeze the eye at the point where the liquid entered the eyeball - if the retina looked attached enough. If not, he would delay the freezing procedure until the retina was healed enough to take on the additional work.

I was sent home to resume my position of humility. It was sort of tough watching TV with my head down, but after some practice, I was able to raise my eyebrows enough to watch my favorite shows by looking at the TV at an upward angle. After another two days, I went back for another check on my progress. To my surprise and realizing that my standings with the Heavenly Head Cheese were solid, my vision test had improved to 20 - 40! Let me just put in a plug here for my doctor, Dr. Hau. He is (No pun intended) a true visionary in the field of visual correction.

Over a period of several weeks, I returned to see Dr. Hau, who performed a series of laser treatments on my eye. Realizing that the part of the eye inside the eye ball really doesn't contain pain receptor cells, the inner eye itself cannot experience much pain. On the other hand, the area around the eye can be very sensitive. The cornea is also very sensitive to pain – have you ever had sand in your eye or scratched your cornea? So, let's just agree that the eye, and the tissue around the eye is sensitive to significant pain when injured. This would also apply to laser treatments. When I got laser tagged, I would sit in the chair – the same type of chair used for any regular eye examination. I never got a good look at the laser equipment, but what I do remember is that Dr. Hau would have me sit very still while he would take hold of my head with one hand, and with the other, he held a device that shot very warm and very bright pulsating strobes into my eye. He would do these series of strobes for around ten to fifteen minutes, pausing on occasion to allow me to rest a bit before blasting me again and again. The best way I can explain how it felt is to say that I felt a lot of pressure – sort of like having a migraine behind your eye. And the light was very hot and bright, causing my eye to gush tears. I would try to relax and try to figure out how many more laser blasts I would get during each session, and I would do my best to relax and think about other things, but the only thing I could really do is to sit still and try not to move and act like a man, when all the while, I was crying buckets!

I can't remember how many laser treatment sessions I had, but I would guess it to be around seven or eight. In between visits, there were days when I saw some big "floaties" in my field of vision. These cobweb-like little creatures would float around a while, change shapes, and disappear then reappear all the time, so that I got used to them – even though it was weird to be looking through a shattered mirror all the time. At least I no longer had to have surgery on my eye, where they actually go into the eye and reattach the retina through another procedure that would be considerably riskier! This procedure, I am told is both painful and a big hassle, since you have to wear a patch and you can't see out of this eye at all for several weeks.

By this time. I was feeling sorry for myself because I was not able to go to Florida, and I was getting tired of going back for "just one more" laser treatment – which happened more than just one more time! But after about three weeks, my eye was healed and my vision had progressed to test at pre-detached retina levels.

But just when things started to look up (excuse the pun), on the morning after the last laser treatment, I woke up to see a dark cloud in front of my other eye!

I had come into the office so many times by then, I was addressing the entire staff on a first name basis and the office I used for treatments had the room number taped over with first aid tape and had words written on the tape that said, "Jim LeDuc's Room." I think they had also considered naming the vision building the Jim LeDuc Retinal Detachment Memorial Building, or something like that, so that when I returned for round two, everyone was pleased to see me1 I suppose that since we had become so close (You may or may not be aware that there is some degree of bonding going on between doctor and staff and patient, during the entire retinal re-attachment process), that everyone appeared to be shocked and concerned and baffled by my other retina following suit so quickly. However, they (nor I) couldn't hide their excitement – our excitement - resulting from our reunion when I returned for round number two!

And so, I went through the whole process again, only this time, instead of receiving laser treatments, the reattachment of this retina was done through a series of treatments using liquid nitrogen! Yes, that is what I said – LIQUID NITROGEN!

I thought that I would need to sign a waiver form which would state that if my eye were to fall out and shatter as it struck the ground, I could not sue for damages! But I signed no such waiver. In fact, these treatments were very similar to the laser – except that there was no bright light. I still felt the pressure, and I was still very uncomfortable during each and every session, but the liquid nitrogen worked just as well. And, I also had a gas bubble injected into this eye as well, but at least until both dissipated over time, I could watch TV through my exclusive 2-D Bubble Vision! (Whatever that means!) I am not sure why the change of treatments, but I think it was due to the fact that my first retina tear was worse than the second, so the welding of my retina back onto the back of the eyeball was not necessary on my second eye. Instead of welding, Dr. Hau felt that freezing the eye back into place was the more effective treatment. Once again, he was correct!

Finally, after a month of liquid nitrogen, and another month of light-pulsating lasers, both my retinas were re-attached, and my vision was restored to its old self. Yes, it's true that I missed going to Orlando with my grandkids, but according to Dr. Hau, it could have been a lot worse – especially if I were over 2500 miles from home when the detachment occurred, and immediate care would be critical, but highly unlikely, as I would have had to get an immediate flight home, and we all know how likely that is! Just think if it were necessary for me to have both eyes operated on, while I did my best impression of Matrix Grandpa Warrior! In the end, I would have to say that my recovery was a miracle! I received immediate care by one of the best eye doctors in the world, and now with over a year past since these procedures, my vision is stable, with no reoccurring symptoms or negative side effects.

Now, here is the lesson part. As you know, my family – my wife, my kids and grandkids – all went to Orlando Florida for a week of vacationing and doing the Disney World stuff. I was not able to make it - of course. Now remembering back when I had my second knee replacement, I asked the doctor how long I should wait until I could fly in an airplane. He told me three months to avoid potential blood clots. Well, I had decided to go to Florida after two months. The doctor seemed a bit concerned I was going, so he told me that if I did go, I needed to reassure him that while I was on the airplane, I would keep moving my leg and get up and walk around frequently.

So now that I am able to reflect on that entire series of events which has now been over a year ago, I believe without a doubt that there was some divine intervention on my part to spare me from getting blood clots and possibly dying. I was given counsel, I fudged on the counsel because I wanted to go to Florida, and the Lord "helped me" do the right thing and save what I believe could have been a catastrophic outcome. That, or it was just a big coincidence…Yeah, right!

Hammertoe

What in thee hell is Hammertoe? How did it get that name? Did someone originally hit their toe with a hammer, so that it became so deformed as to need to be repaired by a doctor, who figured that the only way he or she could fix the now deformed toe would be to strike the toe a second time with a hammer to straighten it out? I have no idea.

A reputable on-line source gives the following information on hammertoe:

A hammer toe is a deformity that causes your toe to bend or curl downward instead of pointing forward. This deformity can affect any toe on your foot. It most often affects the second or third toe. Although a hammer toe may be present at birth, it usually develops over time due to wearing ill-fitting shoes, such as tight, pointed heels, or arthritis. In most cases, a hammer toe condition is treatable.

What Causes a Hammer Toe to Form?

Your toe contains two joints that allow it to bend at the middle and bottom. A hammer toe occurs when the middle joint becomes dislocated.

Common causes of this joint dislocation include:

- a traumatic toe injury
- arthritis
- an unusually high foot arch
- wearing shoes that don't fit properly
- tightened ligaments or tendons in the foot

- pressure from a bunion, which is when your big toe points inward toward your second toe
Spinal cord or peripheral nerve damage may cause all of your toes to curl downward.

As I review this information to see how it relates to my condition. I see some familiar ground. First, I wear a size 15 shoe. Actually, I have wide feet, so I should wear a size 14 wide. However, as I shop for Nike shoes in a wide size, and I almost always wear Nikes every day, I rarely find a wide size. In fact, of all the Nikes I own right now, and I must have at least 40 pair (You might think I have an obsessive-compulsive tendency and you may very well be right, but I am not going to go there just yet!), I have only one pair of wide Nikes. So, I have to buy one size larger, or a size 15, in order for my Nikes to fit. I suppose that this would apply in the bulleted point of "wearing shoes that don't fit properly."

Other possible contributors to my hammertoe are that I have a high arch and I also have arthritis. As a result, my pinky toe on my left foot, which by the way is a half size smaller than my right foot, became deformed so that the bone in the toe began to point outward instead of inward. Because of this, over time a fluid cyst formed in the joint of my pinky toe that would get aggravated every time I wore shoes, to the point where I was teaching my classes in stocking feet!

I went to the podiatrist, another great doctor by the way, and after a quick examination, he informed me that I would need surgery. He explained that the surgical procedure would go as follows: First, he would cut an approximate five-inch long incision along the side of my foot. Once that was done, he would remove the cyst, then cut the bone inside my foot that connected to my toe, he would rotate it so that it was pointing inward instead of outward, then secure it with two very small screws. He told me that I would not be able to put any weight on my foot for about seven weeks, so that as the bone healed and the bone calcified, the screws would be fused inside the bone. He said that my insurance covered crutches (I already have several pairs), but that I would need to purchase my own knee scooter.

And so, that is what he did. The surgery went as planned. My toe was hammered back into place – figuratively speaking – and I was left with the inability to put weight on my foot for weeks. Because my doctor told me that if I were to put any weight on my foot, there was a strong possibility that the screws would not fuse with the bone and the procedure would need to be re-performed, with the likelihood of complications and the probability of a complete recovery to be much lower. So, I followed the doctor's orders. I stayed off my feet and I either used crutches for short distances like to the bathroom, or for long distance travel after three weeks, I used my knee scooter.

Now if you have never seen a knee scooter, it has four wheels and a pad where you can rest the knee of the afflicted foot while you scoot with your good foot. There are several different styles, and I chose the one with the larger wheels for greater stability and built for larger people. I decided not to get the "all-terrain model, since I had no plans of going off-roading while convalescing! The scooter worked quite well and since my classroom was a good distance from where I parked my car, and downhill at that, I enjoyed my morning ride to class! However, along the concrete path to my room, the sidewalk has spaces or seams, which were formed when they poured each section of concrete. Some of these seams, had a fairly nice sized gap of an inch or more, which, when hit by the front tires of the knee scooter, can cause the front end of the scooter to wobble sideways, causing quite a jolt!

After several almost wipeouts going about twenty-five downhill, I made two firm decisions. First, when going downhill, I would always apply the handbrake and keep my speed down to a manageable level by using the hand brake, and second, when going downhill in this seam zone, I would always keep my good foot about an inch above the ground so that I could use my shoe as a secondary brake, just in case I hit a rough spot and started to wobble to the point of wiping out. I made this decision quickly after a few downhill classroom runs, when I kept my good foot too high above the ground, so that it would take about a second too long to lower that good foot down to the sidewalk to apply brakes. In that split second of lowering my shoe to the ground as a secondary brake, I found the wobbling to be unnerving to the point of drooling and showing a facial expression of sheer terror – all while more than a few students looked on in complete delight, cheering me on in hopes of a high-impact, bloody and bone shattering wipe-out!

One other inconvenience with the scooter was the realization that what goes down must then go back up. In other words, I rode the scooter downhill to my class every morning, but that meant that every afternoon, it was necessary for me to ride the scooter back up the hill! However, every cloud has a silver lining as they say, so the advantage to this uphill sojourn was that I was getting in a good workout every day – even when I couldn't stand on two feet to exercise!

Well, I survived the seven weeks and the foot healed completely! The foot did swell on me for at least a month and especially on long days with lots of standing, but after that, I had no further problems. Now that about eight months have passed since the surgery, I can now wear all my shoes without any discomfort or swelling. The results are well worth the temporary inconvenience of travel by scooter.

One More Thing: OCD? Really?!!!

Since the whole point of this book is being honest in my dealings with health issues, I reluctantly need to bring up one more slight health condition that I am developing as I get older. I seem to be having more and more issues with obsessive-compulsive tendencies!!! It's true! I'll be damned if it isn't true! And I never had this problem like I do now! Yes, I have counted my steps on occasion and yes, I have always turned around and clicked my car alarm a second time – even when I absolutely – positively knew that I had already locked the doors before! But over the last several years, I start to get these obsessive thoughts that will not go away, or even diminish – even just a little – until I perform the compulsive act to satisfy that damn obsessive thought!

Let me share a few examples. I have always been a collector of sorts. If you ask my wife, she will tell you that I am a hoarder! It started with knives. As a young boy, I was fascinated by the little black, bone-handled pocket knife that my grandpa always carried around. I remember asking him if I could hold the knife. After reviewing some safety tips, he would let me hold it. I can still remember opening the long blade and feeling it lock into place. His knife had three different blades – one just as sharp as the other as my grandpa would tell me. As I got older, and I began to earn some play money from coaching at high school, I began to collect pocket knives. Over a period of time, my collection expanded. After watching Braveheart for the first time, I knew that I had to get the Claymore sword that William Wallace wielded on the battlefield. This collection went on to include other classic movie swords, like those from 300, Troy, Pirates, The Last Samurai, Lord of the Rings, King Arthur and Gladiator, to name some of the more notable swords. My collection was further enhanced with Bowie knives. I mean, come on! Sylvester Stallone! You just had to come out with The Expendables, and then you had the audacity of creating a script that called for three designer Bowie knives! I had to buy those!

And of course, one simply could not have a knife collection without including Bowie knives with handles made out of antlers, but not just deer antlers, but also water buffalo and ram's horn, could one? And then, there are all the different handle materials, and colors of handles! There's wood and bone and synthetics and metals and carbon fiber, AND there is purple and blue and green and yellow and white and black and so on and so forth. So, before you know it, or before I knew it, I now have a collection of literally hundreds and hundreds of pocket knives, Bowie knives and swords!

I have a bonus room in my house where I have an LCD projector and a big screen where I watch my manly movies with tough guys who use knives and swords of all kinds, so I needed to hang a bunch of movie posters in the room and hang the swords and knives from those movies next to the posters. I have run out of wall space and all I have left is the ceiling but that is where my wife has put her foot down and told me that we are not going to hang weapons of war off of the ceiling! She even went so far as to say that it is time to take down all my knives and swords because we have young grandchildren who could get hurt! She would have me dismantle my man cave – piece by piece – and turn it into a romper room for our grandchildren! **Can you imagine that?!**

Now you might defend me by saying that I just enjoy this collection and there is nothing wrong with having a passionate hobby – Right? Well, if knives were the only "collection" of mine, that would be one thing, but, I do have several other items that I enjoy, no, I am compelled to collect.

My next little obsession is that I love wrist watches! I have one for every occasion. I have sport watches and dress watches. I have a watch in every color of the rainbow and I have a variety of bracelets and leather watch bands. I like the big watches! By big I mean a watch that measures over 50 millimeters across the face of the watch. For me, these fit nicely, and I can get away with a watch that for a smaller person would look more like them strapping a wall clock onto their wrist! Because I own several watch repair kits, I keep the costs down by sizing my watches and by replacing the batteries myself. And, some of my watches are self-winding, so they never need batteries!

Of course, I must mention my considerably large collection of shoes. Nike shoes and Doc Marten dress shoes. I have so many shoes that I have two shoe racks in the master bedroom bath tub! My wife thinks that is excessive! Go figure! I have over forty pairs of Nikes and five or six pairs of Doc Martens.

Then, there are my pens. I like nice pens! I don't have three or four nice pens, I have probably 25 (give or take) pens. Then, there are my neckties. I only wear a tie on Sundays and special occasions. But, I recently found a silk tie hot spot on eBay that sells silk ties for around four dollars. And a lot of them come with cuff links and a pocket square hanky! How can you beat that?

All these culminate in another obsession that I have and that is I feel compelled to match what I am wearing. This means that I need to match colors with shoes, pants, shirts and watches! And believe me, I really doubt I could make it to my car anymore if everything I wore – at least on the outside – did not match! This includes that I would never wear say one shade of teal – like green teal – as the color of my pants, then wear a slightly different shade of teal – like a blue teal – on my shirt or shoes! No Sir-ee Bob! Everything has to match! And just to make sure that I am right with what I wear every day, I lay out what I am going to wear the night before. That way, I can get dressed quickly and get out the door, so I can get to work early. Every once in a while, I feel compelled to change what I am wearing on the morning of…, but most of the time, I am good with my decision from the night before. And usually if I do change the next morning, I have woken up during the night at least once, THINKING about the change! I know, I know…OCD!

One last OCD quirk I have is that when I need to buy toothpaste or lotion or deodorant, I have a strong urge to buy two at a time, "instead of just one, like "normal" people. For some unexplained reason (other than I have these little OCD tendencies), I have this strong urge to always have a backup on hand. If I don't, I get anxious!

This OCD thing seems to have progressed, not from month to month, but over a period of years. As I look back over the past ten years, I can definitely see a trend of becoming more and more compulsive in my buying habits. But luckily, my little obsessions only last a year or so (The knives lasted a decade, but hey! There are lots of knives and swords out there!). After about a year or so, my urges seem to pacify so that I only have one obsession going on at a time. Even that seems a bit on the weird side!

What's Next?

With another several chapters written in the annals of my medical history, I look in the mirror and ask myself, "What's next?" Actually, I try to avoid looking in the mirror for obvious reasons! In fact, when I look at myself – the image of what I truly look like in my sixtieth year of existence – in the mirror, I ask myself, "Who in the hell is that old person in the mirror?! It certainly can't be me!" There are far too many wrinkles and gray hairs and battle scars of life for me to even accept that that image is truly me! Needless-to-say, I avoid mirrors at all cost – just as Count Dracula avoids mirrors. The only difference is that Dracula's reflection cannot be seen by others, while my image cannot be hidden to me or anyone encountering this monster that looks back from the house of mirrors! And as everyone seems to be saying now – and I think that it is the dumbest phrase in the history of the English language – "It is, what it is!" This ridiculously stupid saying is so completely moronic and so obvious and yet, people say it all the time now! Of course, IT IS WHAT IT IS!

From here, I take one day at a time. I look at my calendar right now and I am happy! There are no scheduled procedures or surgeries on the immediate horizon! My back is sore, and I will deal with chronic back pain for the rest of my life. But, since my legs are now straightened out with the aid of titanium, my back feels better. And, because my legs are better, I am exercising fifty minutes a day, five days a week. And, because I am exercising, I am keeping my weight in check and my cholesterol is down to a normal range. So, all in all, my health for the moment is pretty damn good! And that is the best that I can hope for!

So until I add my next couple of chapters, I enjoy life! I do my best at work, I spend time with my wife and kids, and I continue to spoil my grandkids. And every once-in-a-while, I treat myself to a DQ Blizzard!

At this stage of my life, once again I refer to a real good movie to find my new motto of life. It comes from one of Tom Hanks's greatest films, Cast Away. Toward the end, as the main character played by Tom Hanks, Chuck Noland (For which Hanks won an academy award for best actor) reflects back on his life when he was all alone on a very remote island, he says this, and I quote:

"I know what I have to do now. I gotta keep breathing. Because tomorrow the sun will rise. Who knows what the tide could bring?"

And you know what, it just might bring me a sail!

As I close this chapter and keep my mind open to another couple of chapters down the road, I look back through all the medical challenges I have had, and I recognize that I have received excellent treatment, and here I am, still standing – still walking – still elliptical-ing, and I come to a final conclusion. This conclusion comes from a quote from the lyrics of a song by one of the great Rock and Roll artists of my generation, Joe Walsh:

"Life's been good to me so far..."

Made in the USA
Middletown, DE
25 September 2023

38898803R00151